Kettlebells for Sport, Strength and Fitness

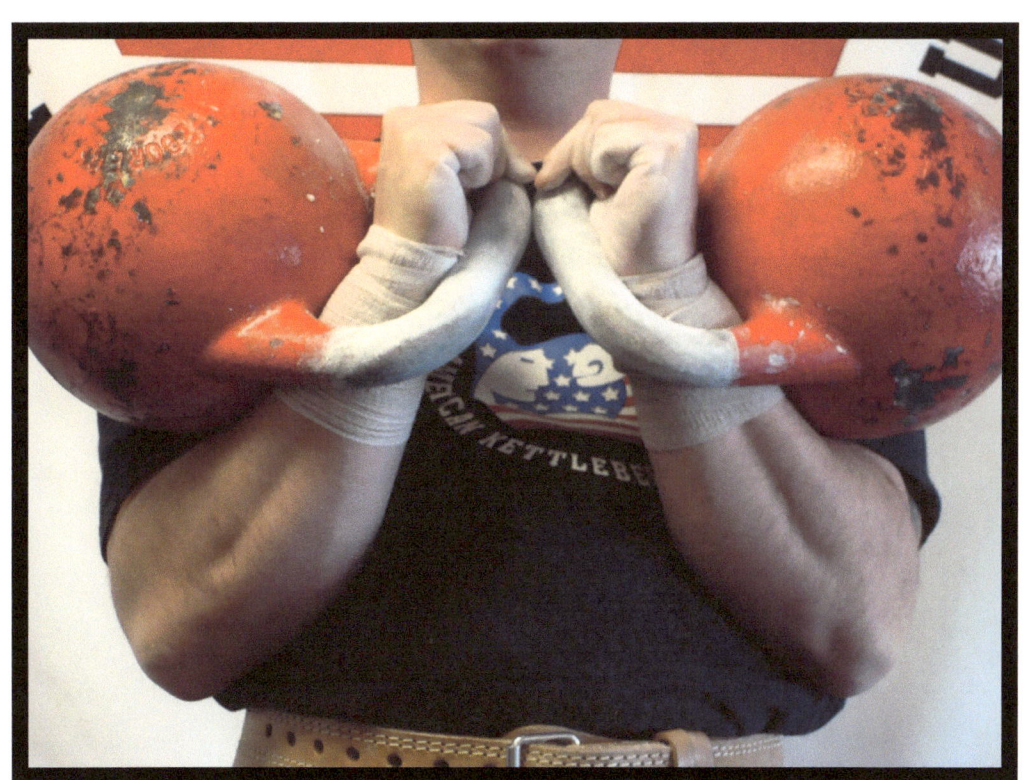

Scott Shetler

Kettlebells for Sport, Strength and Fitness

Scott Shetler

Copyright © 2008 Scott Shetler

ISBN 978-0-615-26229-1

All rights reserved.
No part of this book may be reproduced without the expressed written permission of Scott Shetler.

Published by:
Scott Shetler Performance Training Systems, LLC
2683 Timberbrooke Place
Duluth, GA 30097

Printed in the United States of America.

Visit us on the web at: www.extreme-fitness.org

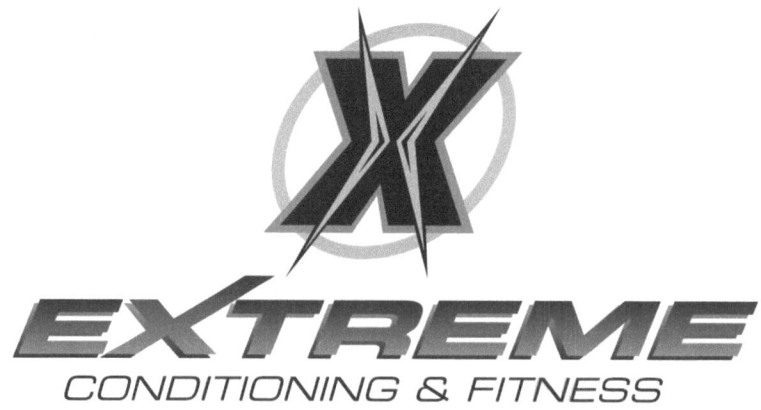

DISCLAIMER: Before beginning any exercise program consult your physician. The author and publisher of this book disclaim any liability, personal or professional, resulting from the misapplication of any of the training procedures described in this publication.

Acknowledgements

I would like to extend a very special thanks to Diane Robert and Flora Health for all of their help and support.

Over the past few years I have been fortunate to meet, train with, and learn from some of the best kettlebell trainers in the USA including Dave Randolph, Steven Mosley, Steve Cotter, Ken Blackburn, Andrew Durniat, Joey Troup, Catherine Imes, and Steve Maxwell. Thank you all for your time, instruction, and friendship.

I would like to extend a special thanks to Valery Fedorenko of the American Kettlebell Club and World Kettlebell Club for offering to teach the methods of kettlebell training that he used to eventually become a world champion and achieve the title of honored master of sport. I would also like to thank Valery for the insight and advice he has given me on how to combine his traditional kettlebell methods with the methods of strength training and sport preparation that I use with my clients and athletes.

Thanks to Eric Liford and Jon Hoskins of the AKC and WKC. Eric has been patient through countless emails of mine and answering many questions that I've sent his way regarding kettlebells and how to best incorporate them into my program. I have always thought that Jon is one of most underrated kettlebell lifters in the US, his technical expertise and performance of the traditional kettlebell lifts is superb.

Of course, thanks to Marty Farrell. Marty was the first American male to achieve the rank master of sport in the sport of kettlebell lifting. I've been friends with Marty for over five years now and watched his struggle from the beginning when he decided to pursue the sport of kettlebell lifting. Marty has taught me a lot, not only about kettlebell training but in the perseverance needed to accomplish your goals.

Thank you all for your friendship and inspiration!

Contents

Preface	5
Chapter 1 – History of Kettlebells	7
Chapter 2 – The Basics	10
Chapter 3 – Kettlebell Exercises	18
Chapter 4 – Training Templates	46
Conclusion	61
About the Author	63
References	64

Preface

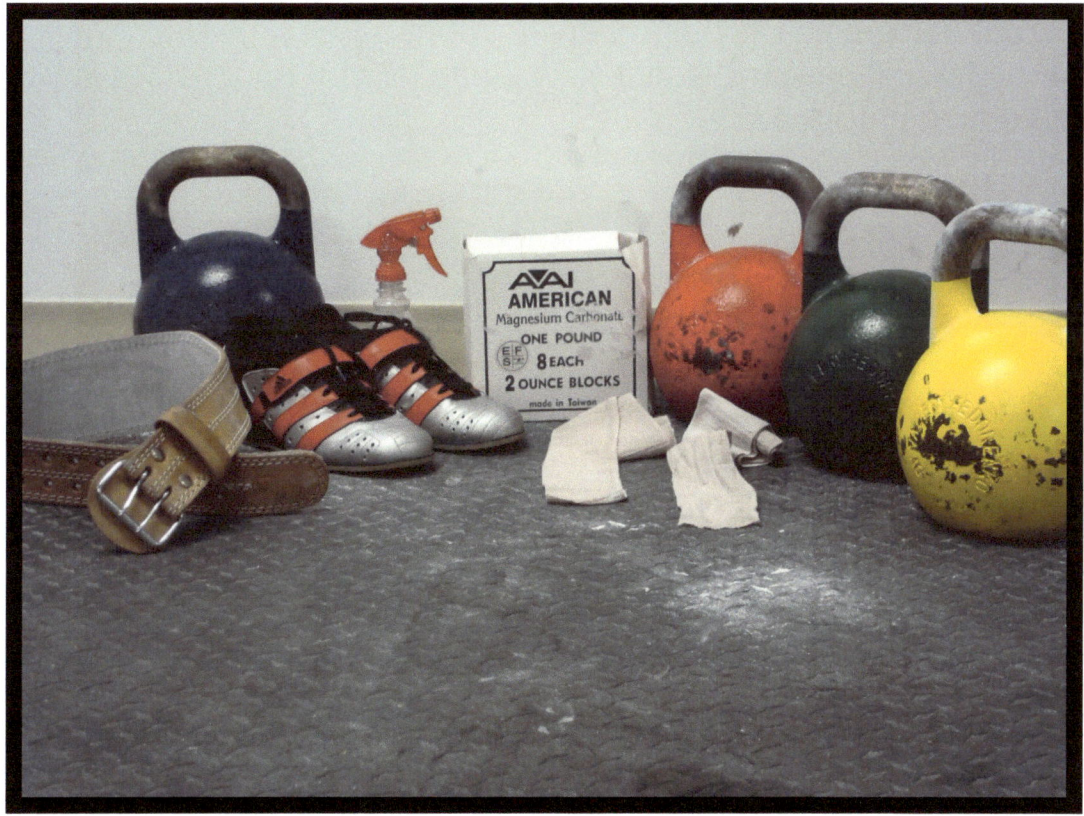

This book deals with kettlebells and how they may be applied to various types of training programs. Whether you are a kettlebell purist or you are looking for a tool that will build your general physical preparation for sport, this book will offer something useful.

In the upcoming chapters you will find information relating to the background of the kettlebell training methods presented, exercise descriptions, important technical pointers, and plenty of sample templates whether your goal is general fitness or sports performance. I have also included personal templates from many of the athletes I train who have benefited from the addition of various forms of kettlebell work in their personal programs.

By no means am I suggesting that this book be considered the be-all, end-all of kettlebell training. Rather it is my sincerest hope that you approach these methods with an open-mind and understand that what I am presenting is based on my personal experience and limited to the scope of my practice with these valuable training tools.

With that being said I hope you enjoy the material presented in this book and that it presents some new ideas for you to consider in your own training program.

Chapter 1
History of Kettlebells

Kettlebells have been used for hundreds of years. Originally they were used as units of measure by farmers in Russia and Eastern Europe. Around the end of the XVII century, kettlebells in weights of 16kg, 32kg and 48kg were used for a show of strength at different holidays, fairs and later in circuses.

Anyone familiar with turn-of-the-century physical culture will know that old-time strongmen used kettlebells, or ring-weights, quite often in their exercise programs. A Google search on names like Arthur Saxon, Eugene Sandow, and Sig Klein will reveal many documents and pictures of these men performing feats of strength with various types of kettlebells and ring-weights.

In 2007 my wife and I made the journey to the Weightlifting Hall of Fame in York, PA while on vacation, and I was surprised to see different styles of kettlebells on display in some of the display cases. There were German kettlebells and ring-weights of different sizes and styles.

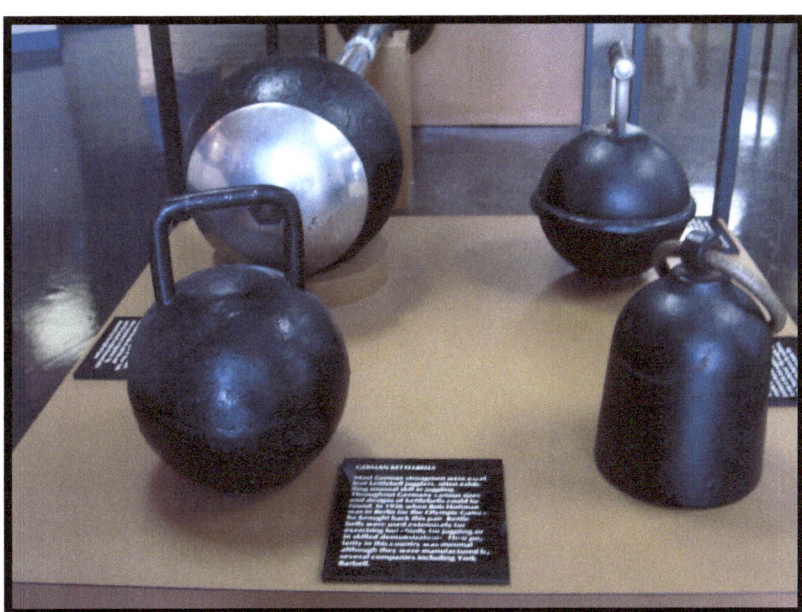

Kettlebells & Ring-Weights displayed at the Weightlifting Hall of Fame in York, PA

Around 1948, the sport of kettlebell lifting emerged. While there were no structured rules or sport classification system, competitions became more organized and typically events utilizing 32kg kettlebells prevailed. By 1962 the sport became even more organized in that rules and sport classifications were developed.

Originally the lifts contested were the one-arm snatch, one-arm press, and the two-arm jerk. This sport differed from weightlifting in that the fixed weight kettlebells were lifted for repetitions over a set time period, whereas in weightlifting the athlete lifted a maximal weight for one repetition.

Eventually the press was taken out of kettlebell sport competition and to this day the biathlon consists of the one-arm snatch and two-arm jerk. Repetitions between the two lifts are added together to produce the athlete's total score.

A second competition was later added which became its own event, a two-arm clean and jerk referred to as the long cycle. In the long cycle clean and jerk two kettlebells are cleaned to the chest then jerked overhead. At this point the bells are lowered to the chest and then re-cleaned for the next repetition.

Women typically compete in the one-arm snatch only, although in some organizations this is changing and women are performing a one-arm biathlon and one-arm long cycle as well.

While these are the more traditionally contested lifts it is common to see other events at competitions. Lifts such as presses, chair presses, one-arm long cycle, and jerk relay events are commonly seen.

Impressive feats of strength are often performed as well. Bottoms up clean and presses, presses done while holding the kettlebell by the pinky finger, deadlifting a kettlebell from the ground by the pinky finger, and different juggling exercises in which athletes toss and flip kettlebells in the air and sometimes to other athletes are some of the more common feats of strength performed with kettlebells.

There is a fantastic online resource **"Caestus: The Extreme Girevoy Sport Records Blog"** that can be found at **caestuspalestra.wordpress.com**. If you want a detailed history of kettlebell sport (also referred to as girevoy sport) as well as numerous blogs and articles about kettlebell lifting, kettlebell lifters, and the history of kettlebell lifting you cannot go wrong with this blog. It is an excellent resource for all things kettlebell-related.

Today kettlebells have found a home in fitness training and exercise right next to barbells and dumbbells. While the sport of kettlebell lifting is growing in popularity, many people are happy enough incorporating kettlebells into their personal fitness regimens. In the US everyone from soccer moms to NFL players are using kettlebells and their popularity continues to grow. Some think they are simply another fitness fad but many believe they are here to stay.

Chapter 2
The Basics

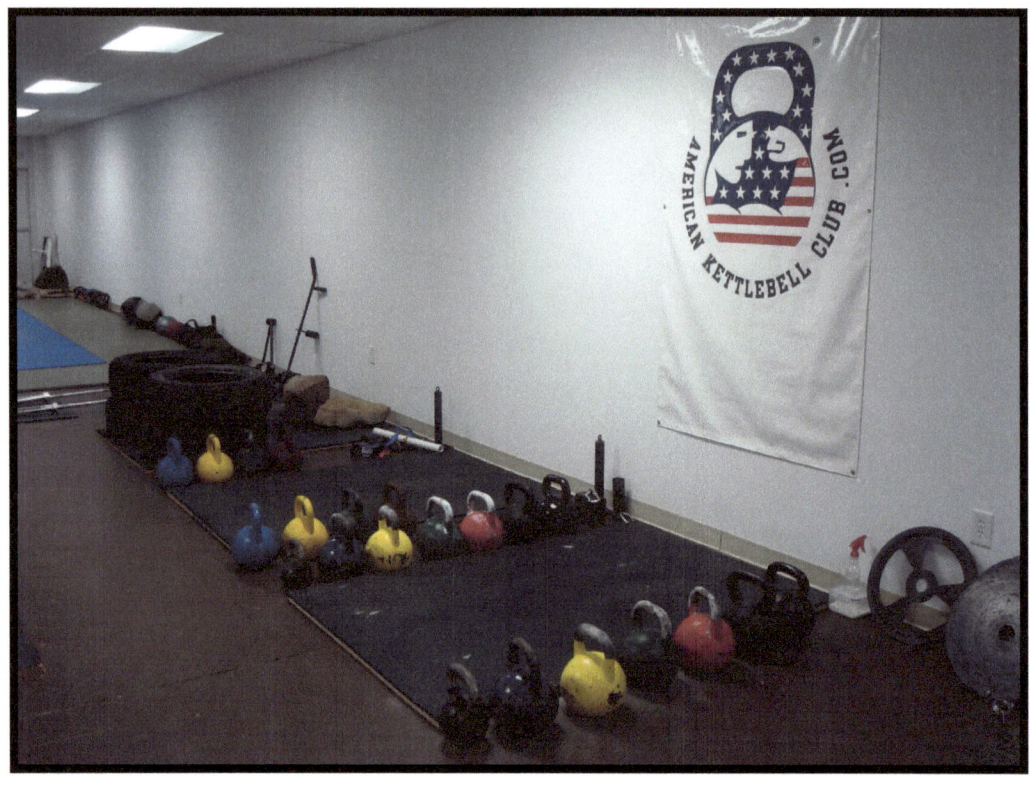

It is virtually impossible to say what kettlebells should or should not be used for. Because they are nothing more than a handle attached to a weighted ball their use is limited to the user's creativity and imagination.

Since kettlebells are fixed weights that traditionally come in odd sizes, there are many who believe that the most effective way to use kettlebells is in the traditional lifts for high repetitions. In my personal training and practice I have found this to be the case.

I honestly believe that for progressive strength training barbells and dumbbells win hands down. They can be loaded incrementally and lend themselves to the strength lifts such as squats, bench press, rows, and deadlifts far better than kettlebells ever could.

I am not saying that you could not grab a kettlebell and do a row with it, I have done plenty of kettlebell rows in my own training, but when it's time to move up in weight, jumping from a 53 pound kettlebell to a 70 pound kettlebell is a much bigger jump than going from a 55 pound dumbbell to a 60 pound dumbbell. Remember, in training pick the best tool for the job!

Kettlebell Styles

There are many different types of kettlebells on the market today. Obviously price is a very important factor when choosing kettlebells and honestly if all you plan to do are swings and maybe an occasional press or snatch most any bell will do.

I have used many different brands of kettlebells myself and favor the **Pro-Grade Kettlebells** available from the **American Kettlebell Club/World Kettlebell Club**. These bells are styled after the kettlebells most often used by Russian and other Eastern European kettlebell lifters.

There are many benefits to using the Pro-Grade kettlebell. One of the biggest reasons is that these bells were specifically designed for kettlebell lifting. They fit very well on the arm in the rack position for jerks and presses. Their design allows them to "lock" perfectly onto the forearm during snatches and in the overhead position in the jerk and press, without crowding the wrist.

The handle is typically between 32-35 millimeters which allows you to utilize the finger-lock grip in swings and snatches allowing you to perform very high repetitions while reducing the chance of tearing the skin on your palm.

Another benefit is that the Pro-Grade bells are all the same dimension regardless of weight. This allows you to use the exact same technique whether you are moving up from the 12kg bell to the 16kg bell or from the 24kg bell to the 32kg bell.

Many of my clients have enjoyed these benefits and began replacing their personal kettlebells with the Pro-Grade kettlebells. Due to the fact that these bells are the same size they are typically color-coded in order to identify different weights quickly. It is standard that 12kg bells are blue, 16kg bells are yellow, 24kg bells are green, and 32kg bells are red.

Sets and Reps

When it comes to sets and reps we use a different approach with kettlebells. I am not saying it is impossible to perform 3 sets of 10 reps with a kettlebell exercise. If you are a first-time kettlebell lifter this may produce results.

However, kettlebells are not that heavy, particularly for the exercises we utilize them for. If they were heavy people would not be performing hundreds of repetitions with them for ten to twenty minutes without setting the bells down.

I know of one American lifter, who does exceptionally well in the long cycle event, and performed over 200 repetitions in the 1-arm long cycle event with a 32kg kettlebell in twenty minutes. He was allowed to switch hands as many times as he chose, although he was not able to set the bell down at any point. This is an awesome feat of strength-endurance in my opinion. A little quick math shows that this is a pace of 10 repetitions per minute.

Give it a shot, put this book down, grab your 32kg bell and perform 1-arm long cycle clean and jerks at a pace of 10 reps per minute for twenty minutes without setting your bell down.

Since I do not favor the traditional bodybuilding set and repetition schemes for kettlebell lifting what do I recommend for sets and repetitions? I favor timed sets without setting the kettlebell down.

Remember, our goal with kettlebells is strength-endurance. If we want absolute strength, power, or muscle hypertrophy we are going lift barbells and dumbbells, which are much better suited for those goals.

Later in this book I will present general templates on utilizing kettlebells by themselves as well as with barbells and dumbbells. I will present some templates I have used with some of my athletes and clients as well.

Timed Sets

There are many benefits to timed sets. Timed sets allow you to build pace for a given period of time. When performing timed sets with a slower pace you will learn the value of building a strong rack or resting position.

Building a strong rest position is very important as we typically prefer to not set the bell down until the set is complete. This keeps the working muscles under tension for the duration of the set. This is something that powerlifting coach Louie Simmons of the Westside Barbell Club in Columbus, Ohio wrote extensively about in his articles detailing the repeated effort method and how he implements timed sets of barbell and dumbbell lifts in his training and the training of his powerlifters.

Keep in mind that timed sets can be one minute, five minutes or even twenty minutes or more.

Kettlebell sport competitions use ten minutes as the limit for the lifts. This does not mean that performing three minute sets is not beneficial. Obviously for competition you will need to perform ten minute sets in training.

If your goal is fitness there is nothing wrong with performing multiple sets of two, three or four minutes. On occasion take a very light bell and try to go twenty minutes or more.

I do a lot of my "competitive" training sets with the 24kg bell but I have found that grabbing the 16kg once a week and performing snatches or 1-arm long cycle at a pace of 12-14 reps per minute, or a combination of both for twenty minutes without setting the bell down has been great for cardiovascular work.

I am usually drenched head to toe in sweat by the end of the set. This is a great way to get some good training in with a very light kettlebell.

The powerlifters that train at my gym regularly perform timed sets of swings, clean and jerks, snatches or presses as "finishers" after their strength work.

Valery Fedorenko recommended that we use something in the ballpark of three minute sets for the powerlifters to help boost their GPP.

One of our lifters decided to try a three minute set for as many reps as possible with 24kg bells in the long cycle following a max effort squat workout and ended up showering the bathroom with the pulled pork sandwich he had for lunch. Yum! He switched to the 16kg bells in his next workout.

For conditioning work the kettlebells do not need to be that heavy. Only once you start hitting the upper limits of the reps per minute at a given weight should you move up to the next size of kettlebell.

Repetitions Per Minute (RPM)

For presses, jerks and long cycle begin with 4 to 5 repetitions per minute. For snatches a pace of 12 to 14 repetitions per minute is usually a good starting point.

It is important to start with a slow pace as it will allow you to build comfort in the rack or resting positions and you will not tire yourself out quickly like you would by beginning with a faster pace.

Due to the lack of a resting component in the swing exercise there is no recommended pace, however you will find when training the swing you will use a pretty consistent tempo every time you do them.

As far as upper limits of pacing are concerned for jerks and snatches it's going to be 24 repetitions per minute, anything faster would not be a complete repetition in which a definitive lockout overhead is demonstrated.

For long cycle it will be around 14 repetitions per minute. Consider the absolute world record performances in the competition lifts at the time of this writing.

For the jerk it is 175 reps in ten minutes with a pair 32kg kettlebells done by Ivan Denisov, for the snatch it is 220 repetitions in ten minutes with a 32kg kettlebell 110 reps per arm with one hand switch done by both Ivan Denisov and Valery Fedorenko, and in the long cycle it is 109 repetitions with two 32kg kettlebells done by Ivan Denisov.

For the jerk Denisov is lifting at a pace between 17 and 18 repetitions per minute, for the snatch he is lifting at a pace of 22 repetitions per minute, and for the long cycle he is lifting at a pace of 11 repetitions per minute.

Lifter Rankings and Classifications

I think it is important to mention a bit about the lifter ranking system for the sport of kettlebell lifting for those of you who are considering participation in the sport.

Lifter rankings or classifications are determined by two things, the lifter's weight class and the total number of repetitions the lifter performs. Russian and Eastern European countries used this system of classification for all athletics.

In the professional ranks a beginner is someone who has achieved a **Class III** ranking. Moving up from beginner level is **Class II** (intermediate), **Class I** (advanced) and **Candidate for Master of Sports** or **CMS** (highly advanced).

After **CMS** ranking is **Master of Sports or MS** (national ranking) and finally **Master of Sports, International Class** or **MSIC** (international ranking).

Above this there is an **Honored Master of Sports**, a title awarded to a sportsman for their achievements and contributions to the sport.

Please note that in the sport of kettlebell lifting, under the rules of the World Kettlebell Club, one can achieve **Class III- MSIC** ranking only by participating in open professional competition.

For men this means competing with the 32kg kettlebells and 16kg kettlebells for the women although at the time of this writing there is discussion of moving professional women up to the 20kg kettlebell.

Amateurs and Master's competitors may achieve **Class VII-IV** ranks with their respective kettlebells, 24kg for men and 12kg for women although the WKC is considering moving amateur men to the 28kg kettlebell and amateur women to the 16kg kettlebell.

The events a lifter may achieve rank in are the biathlon and long cycle for men and the one-arm biathlon for women. Classification standards for the women's one-arm long cycle are currently being developed. If you would like to view the current WKC lifter classification charts please visit their website at **www.worldkettlebellclub.com**.

I should also note, while on the subject of lifter classification rankings, in 2006 the Russian Federation updated their ranking system.

For the men **CMS-MSIC** is achieved in open competition with the 32kg kettlebell and **Class III-I** is achieved with the 24kg kettlebell for the biathlon and long cycle events.

Women can qualify in the snatch-only competition and **Class III-MSIC** rankings are achieved with the 24kg kettlebell.

Traditional vs. Non-Traditional Exercises

Even though I firmly believe in using kettlebells for the traditional lifts in the methods that I learned through Valery Fedorenko and the American Kettlebell Club, I have on occasion used variations of traditional dumbbell exercises with kettlebells and found the kettlebell version to be more effective. I was inspired to try this when I heard of Fedorenko's coach, Pandelis Filikidi, who used very heavy kettlebells for curl exercises to build strength for arm wrestling.

I have experimented with a triceps extension variation with my powerlifters. I have noticed great carryover to the bench press lockout as a result, particularly with David Cohn, my lifter in the 114 and 123 pound weight classes.

When David started training with me he had a personal best of 260 pounds in the bench press at a bodyweight of 111 pounds. We have successfully raised his bench press to 275 pounds at a bodyweight of 111 pounds and recently at the time of this writing made a 305 pound bench at a bodyweight of 120 pounds.

Our special kettlebell extension exercise is part of a regular rotation in David's toolbox of supplementary lifts and I will detail the exercise in the non-traditional kettlebell exercise section of the chapter in this book dedicated to kettlebell exercises.

Please keep in mind it is only in these special situations that I deviate from traditional kettlebell training methods. For the bulk of my trainees, when it comes to kettlebell training, we follow a steady diet of the traditional lifts and methods.

Chapter 3
Kettlebell Exercises

In this chapter I will present the traditional exercises I use in my training and the training of my clients and athletes. I will discuss important technical points in the performance of each lift as well.

Please keep in mind that I am constantly learning, and by no means consider myself an expert in the technical aspects of these lifts. I only hope to share with you what I have learned and retained through my training with Coach Valery Fedorenko and some of the better lifters in the American Kettlebell Club.

As I am always learning and looking for the best possible technique, I encourage you to do the same. This way you are always evolving your training program, learning and experimenting. I believe if you become comfortable in your training your progress will come to a halt.

In addition to the traditional lifts and lifting methods I will share some non-traditional lifts that we have found useful as well. Keep in mind I do not implement traditional or non-traditional lifts in my training or that of my clients for "something neat to do" or to "change things up".

I believe you must be clear and definite in stating your goals. Once your goals are in place, use the most effective and efficient means of getting there. Anything else is a waste of your time, in my opinion.

With that being said, let's take a look at the kettlebell lifts.

Traditional Kettlebell Exercises

Before we actually detail the exercises let's talk about some key points regarding preparation of the handle of the kettlebell as well as how to properly grip the bell for the exercises.

These two important points will help you avoid problems like tearing off calluses or ripping the skin on the palm of your hand during high repetition swings, clean and jerks and snatches.

In addition we will discuss the use of wrist wraps, belts and other methods pertaining to kettlebell lifting such as breathing and building a strong rack position.

Preparation

In order to properly prepare the handle of your kettlebell first ensure that the paint has been completely removed from the handle. If you are purchasing the newer generation of the **American Kettlebell Club/World Kettlebell Club Pro-Grade Kettlebells**, this will not be an issue as they are being shipped with the paint already removed from the handle.

An industrial file can be useful to smooth out any imperfections or rough areas on the handle as well. Once the handle is completely bare apply chalk liberally to the entire handle. Be sure to spend some time and coat the handle well so that the handle remains chalked for the duration of your set.

You will most likely need to reapply chalk for further training sets in the session.

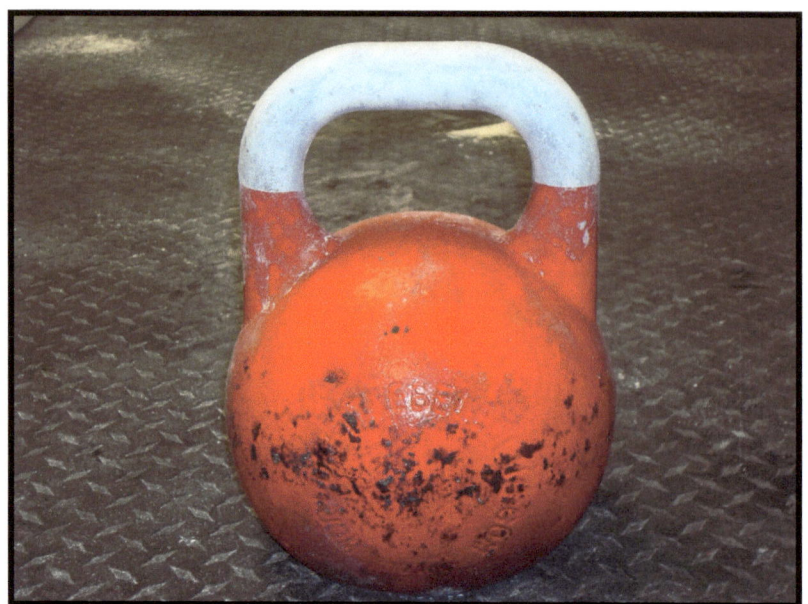
A properly prepared kettlebell

Chalking of the hands is just as important as chalking the handle of the kettlebell. Be sure to cover the entire surface of the palm side of the hand as well as the index finger and thumb. You may want to cover the outside area of the hand between the base of the thumb and base of the index finger.

Additionally some people chalk the backside of the tip of the index finger as this is where the tip of the thumb "locks" the finger on the handle of the bell during swings, cleans and snatches.

In addition to chalking the hands, many lifters use some form of wrist wrap. While this does cushion the wrist and forearm to some extent, the main purpose is to keep the surface of the arm where the bell rests dry. If this area is moist with sweat, the bell may slide out of position very easily. This could result in missed repetitions.

Most lifters use a simple ace bandage cut in half and wrapped around the lower forearm/wrist area. Alternatively some lifters use tennis or basketball style wrist bands as these are quite easy to slide on and off.

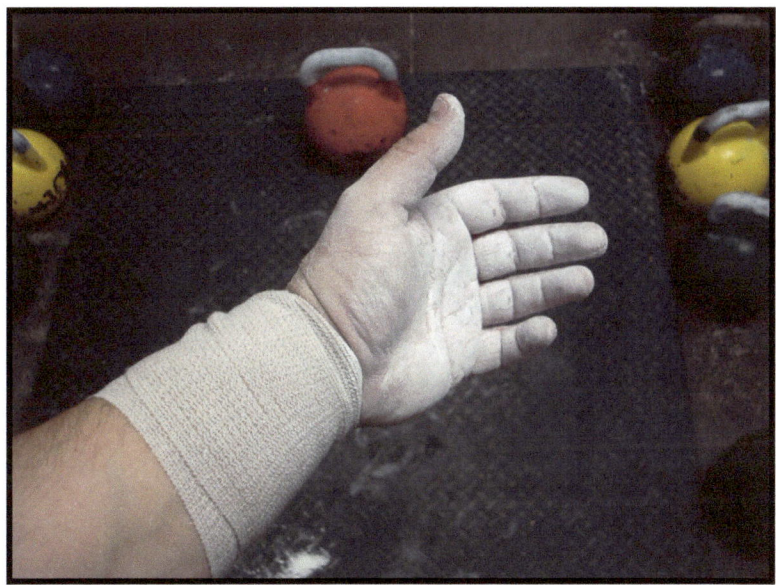
Chalked, wrapped and ready to lift!

Grip

When gripping the kettlebell, the optimal area to hold the bell is on the thumb-side corner of the handle. Then, wrap the index finger and thumb around the handle and lock the grip in place by "trapping" the index finger to the handle with the thumb. We refer to this as the "finger lock" grip. If you are familiar with the hook grip in weightlifting, the finger lock is basically the opposite.

Once applying the finger lock the remaining three fingers are curled around the handle. This grip will be applied to all of the traditional kettlebell exercises.

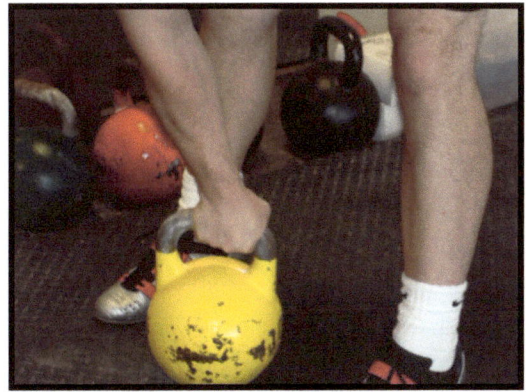
Gripping the Kettlebell

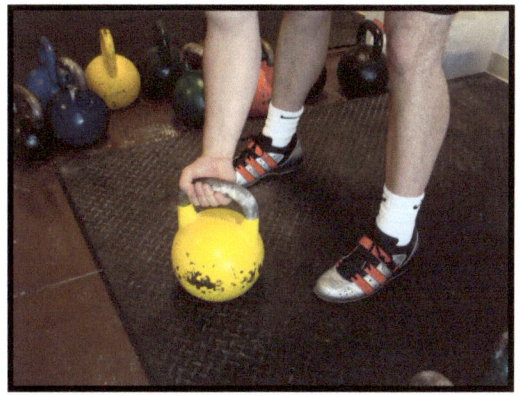
Finger-Lock Technique

21

Belts

Some people choose to use lifting belts while performing the kettlebell lifts. In the sport of kettlebell lifting, it is now illegal to use the belt as a device to rest the elbows on while in the rack position, so there is not much benefit for the lifter. Some people use the belt to keep their shirt tucked in and some just like to "feel" something on their back. Keep in mind that the belts used for kettlebell lifting, the thin belts that are 4" in the back and taper to 2" in the front offer very little, if any, support to the lumbar spine. These are nowhere near as supportive as a 13mm thick, 4" wide powerlifting belt.

Considering the risk of being disqualified due to the elbows touching the belt while in the rack position, it is not worth wearing a belt, in my opinion. If you are not training for kettlebell sport a belt should not be worn period.

If you are looking to "enhance" the rack position you may use a spray bottle to wet each side of your t-shirt where the elbows rest in the rack position. This will allow your elbows to "grab" your shirt and assist in the rack position. Again, this technique is more applicable to the kettlebell sport competitor than someone training for fitness.

Breathing

The breathing pattern in kettlebell lifting is the opposite of the breathing pattern used when lifting a very heavy weight. Kettlebells are relatively light. If they were not, lifters would not perform hundreds of repetitions without setting the bells down to rest.

Since kettlebell lifts are typically performed for high repetitions, thus making kettlebell lifting more of a strength-endurance exercise than an absolute strength exercise, the breathing pattern needs to be different than you would use when lifting a very heavy weight.

When a lifter attempts a very heavy barbell lift, such as the squat, the lifter will typically hold their breath through the entire repetition in order to pressurize the abdominal cavity and support the spine. They may exhale forcefully as they blast through the most difficult phase of the lift to the lockout.

In kettlebell lifting for high repetitions the goal is to conserve energy. The breathing pattern is such that when the bells are lifted up as in the peak of the swing or the snatch, jerk or press overhead, the lifter inhales as the chest cavity opens up and expands. As the bell is lowered and the chest cavity collapses, the lifter will exhale. This is a much more compatible form of breathing with this type of activity.

Rack Position

Before we get into the exercises let's take a minute and go over the rack position. The rack position will be important for many of the lifts and is typically one of the most difficult aspects of kettlebell lifting to perform correctly.

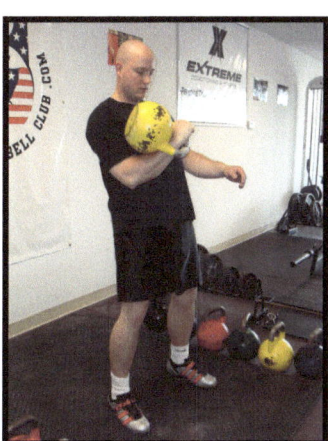
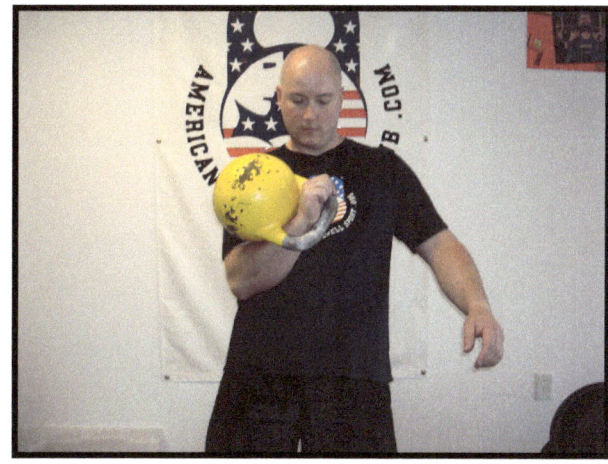

Single-Kettlebell Rack Position

In the rack position the bell is resting between the wrist and the shoulder in the "v" of the arm. In order to maximize the ability to perform higher and higher repetitions it is imperative to build a strong and efficient rack position. This position relies largely on structure rather than muscle. The goal is eventually to be able to rest the elbows on the upper tip of the hip bone. This will allow you to relax as much as possible in between repetitions and prevent fatigue.

The hands are placed near the thumb-side curve of the handle. The pointer finger and thumb are looped around the handle and the remaining fingers are curled back behind the handle. This is mainly to prevent smashing the fingers between the handles when performing two kettlebell exercises.

The handle rests on the heel of the palm near the wrist and the wrist is relaxed but not bent back. The hands are turned with the palms facing each other and slightly turned out.

The hips are pushed forward and the upper back is rounded or hunched forward to facilitate resting the elbows on the hips. The last key point is to keep the knees straight. Allowing the knees to bend will fatigue the quads very quickly.

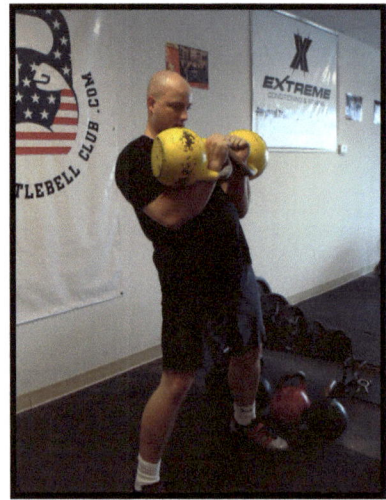 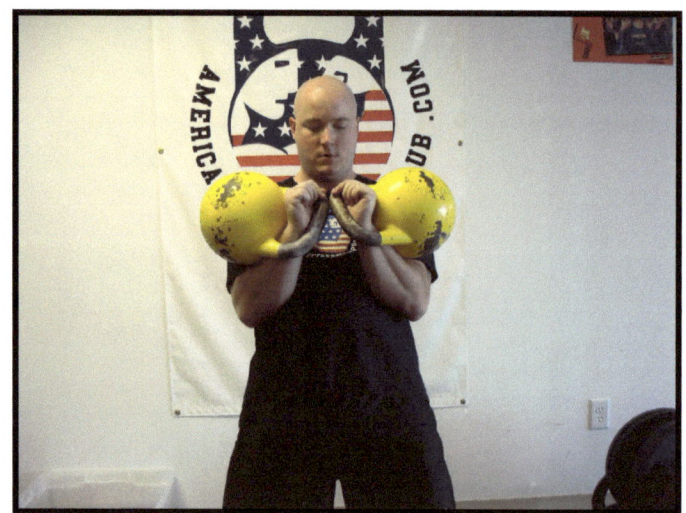

Double-Kettlebell Rack Position

Swing

This swing is probably the most basic exercise in kettlebell lifting. Swings will be the foundation for many of the other kettlebell lifts. In addition swings will teach you to use your entire body as a unit, improve your conditioning and grip, and strengthen your back. The will give you a fantastic opportunity to perfect your breathing techniques as well.

There is a very specific way in which we teach the swing, as this exercise is a foundation exercise for the more advanced kettlebell snatch. Heavy swings are crucial in building the snatch exercise numbers as well.

To begin the exercise pick the bell up and swing it back between the legs, the thumb should be pointing back in the bell's direction of travel during the swing-back phase of the movement. At the end of the swing-back the spine should be in a neutral position, although some rounding in the thoracic spine region (upper back) may occur, which is fine.

Swing the bell up by extending the back and hips and almost shrugging up on the shoulder of the working arm. At this point do not project the bell out in front of you, rather pull up by bending the elbow slightly and allowing the bell to travel in more of a vertical path upward. At the peak of the movement the bell will feel almost weightless. This should occur around the upper abdominal or chest region.

Allow the bell to fall back down on the same path it came up on. Be sure to apply the finger lock grip and allow the bell to completely decelerate before redirecting the movement. This technique will save energy and your grip will not fatigue as quickly. You may even find that the bell travels up in a slight arc at the peak of the swing back.

It may help to think of the swing as a pendulum. It is a very fluid movement. Be sure to think efficiency when performing this exercise. If you try to muscle through it you will not be able to get near as many reps as if you relaxed and performed the exercise in a more efficient manner.

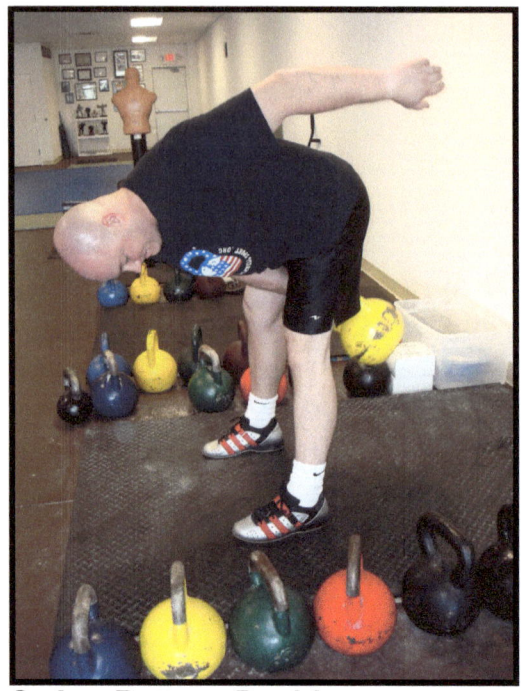 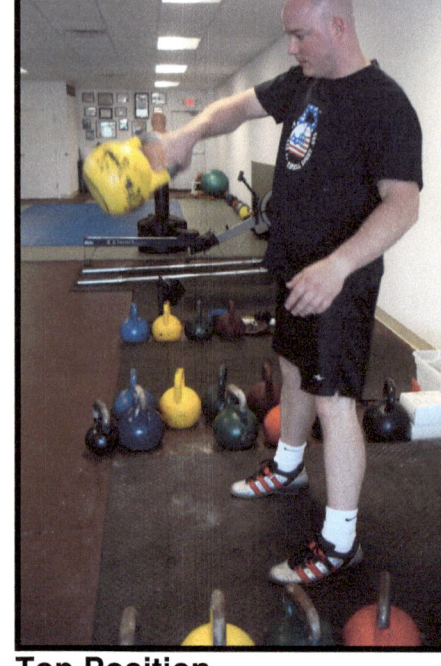

Swing Bottom Position   **Top Position**

Since there is no resting component for swings, there is no recommended repetition per minute (RPM) pace and are typically performed for a set number of repetitions. Swings are a fantastic supplemental exercise in building the snatch and are typically performed with a heavier kettlebell than your snatch weight. For instance, if you are a masters-level competitor using the 24kg kettlebells, performing high repetition swings with the 32kg would be typical. Since we use the swing to build the snatch and need a similar range of motion we only perform swings with one hand.

Primary Muscles Worked

hamstrings, glutes, lower back, upper back, grip

Clean

The clean begins exactly like the swing only instead of pulling the kettlebell up you are actually going to roll it around your hand and arm allowing it to land in the rack position. After catching the bell in the rack position reverse the movement by rolling the bell back around the hand and arm allowing it to swing back between the legs to perform the next repetition.

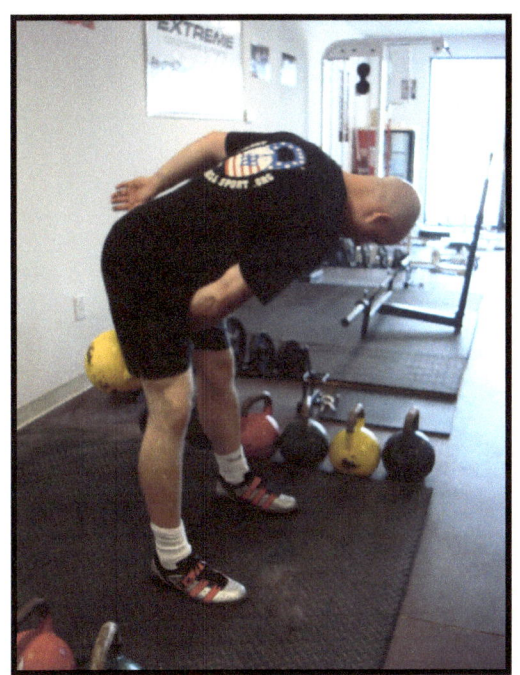
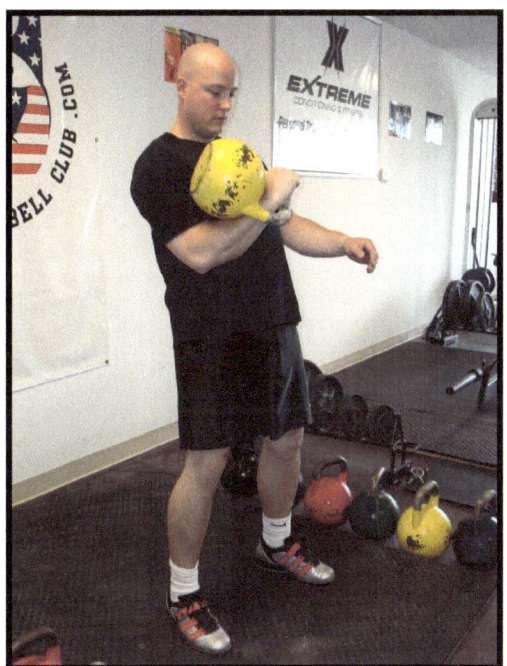

Clean Bottom Position **Catching the Bell in the Rack Position**

In the clean the RPMs will typically range from 4-16 and may be performed with one or two kettlebells.

Variations

Bottom-Up Clean

The bottom up clean is a variation in which the clean is performed only the bell is caught and balanced upside down. This is a great means for improving the strength of the grip and forearms.

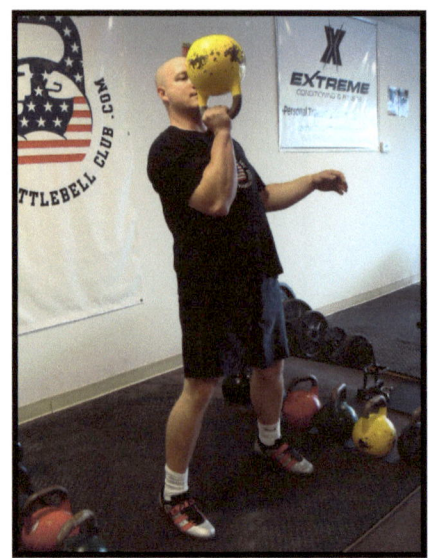

Bottom-Up Clean

Primary Muscles Worked

hamstrings, glutes, lower back, upper back, grip

Press

The press begins in the rack position. In the strict press the knees must remain straight. You may not "hop" the bell up with the knees or ankles to create an initial momentum. From the rack position press the weight straight up and overhead until the arm is completely straight. It is important that the inside of the bicep be near the ear.

Do not let the arm rotate out to the side. Once the bell is fixed overhead in a proper lockout position, reverse the movement and lower the bell back to the rack.

Lowering the bell in a quick but controlled manner is recommended in order to prevent fatigue and achieve higher repetitions.

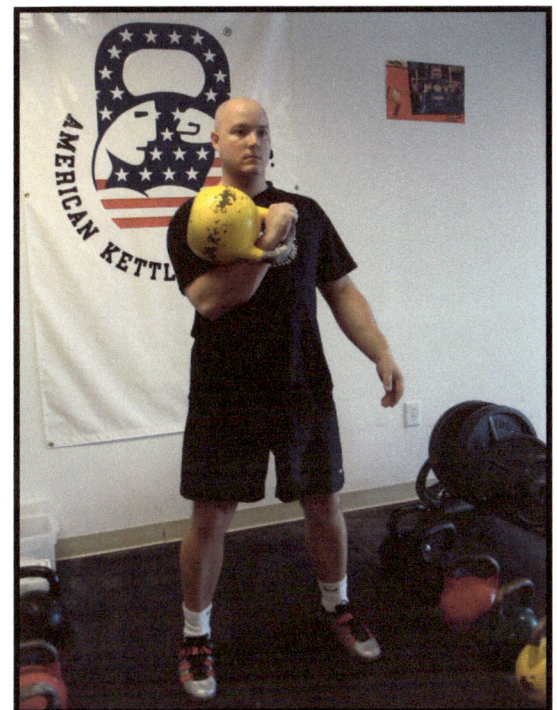 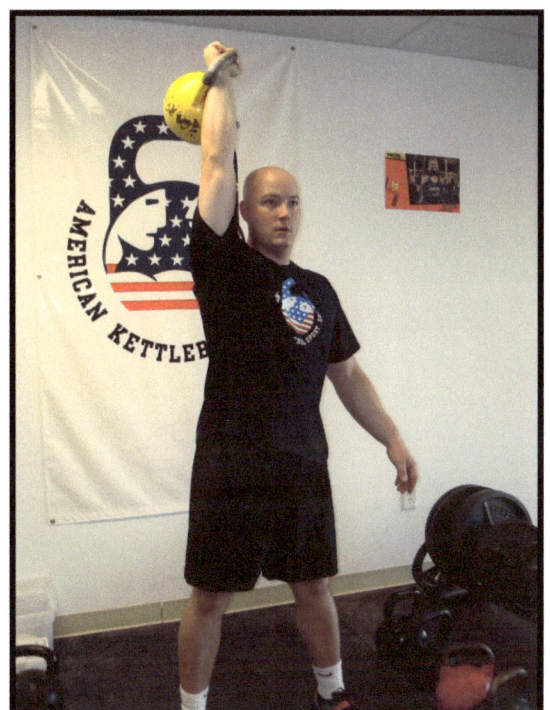

The Press Rack Position **Lockout**

In the press the RPMs will typically range from 4-12. Presses may be performed with one or two kettlebells, although when this was one of the contested lifts it was performed with one kettlebell.

Variations

Bottom-Up Press

The bottom-up press is a variation in which the kettlebell is held and balanced upside down and pressed overhead to a lockout. This stresses the grip and the forearm more than a regular press.

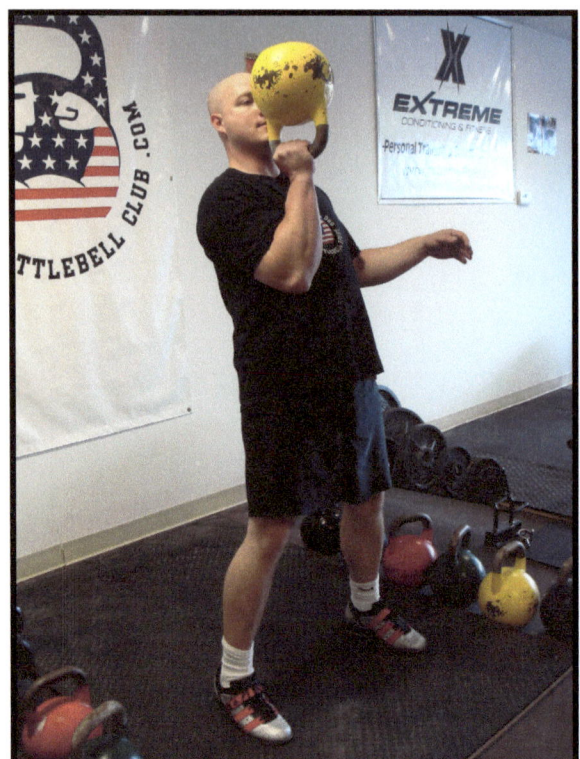
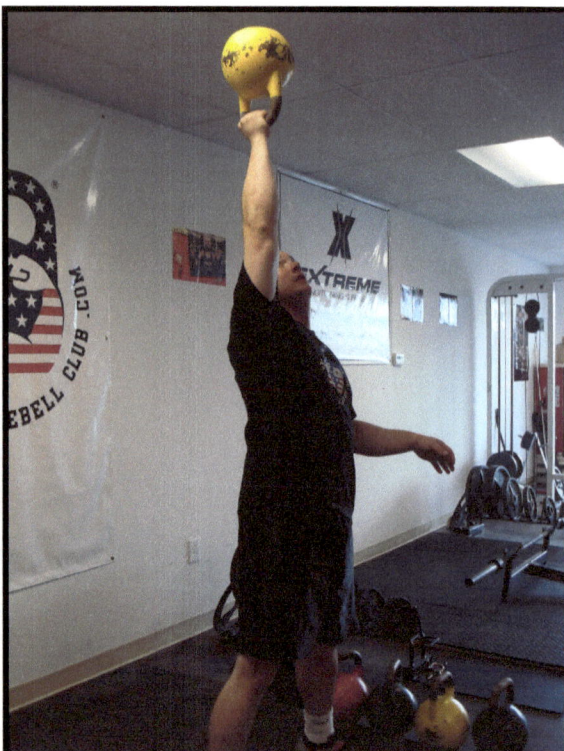

Bottoms-Up Press

Chair Press

The chair press is performed by cleaning the bell to the rack position and sitting on a chair or bench. Once seated, press the bell overhead to a lockout then return to the rack position. The chair press may be performed with one or two kettlebells.

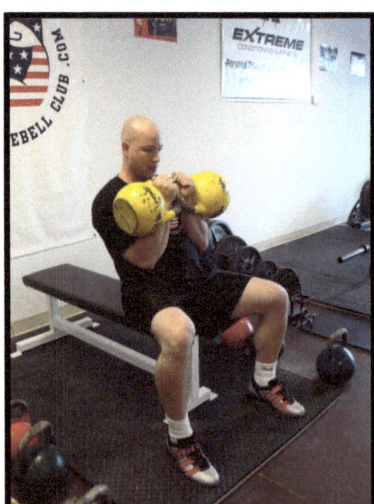
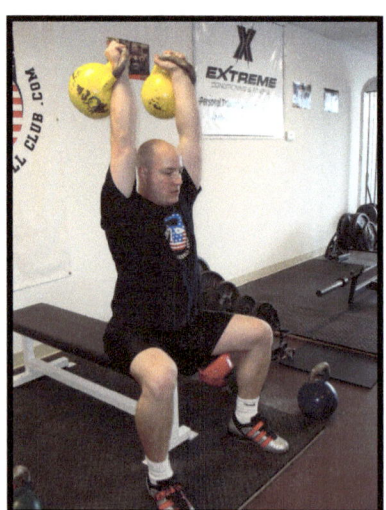

Chair Press

Variations

Bottom-Up Chair Press

Clean the kettlebell(s) into a bottom-up position then sit down onto the bench or chair and perform the press exercise.

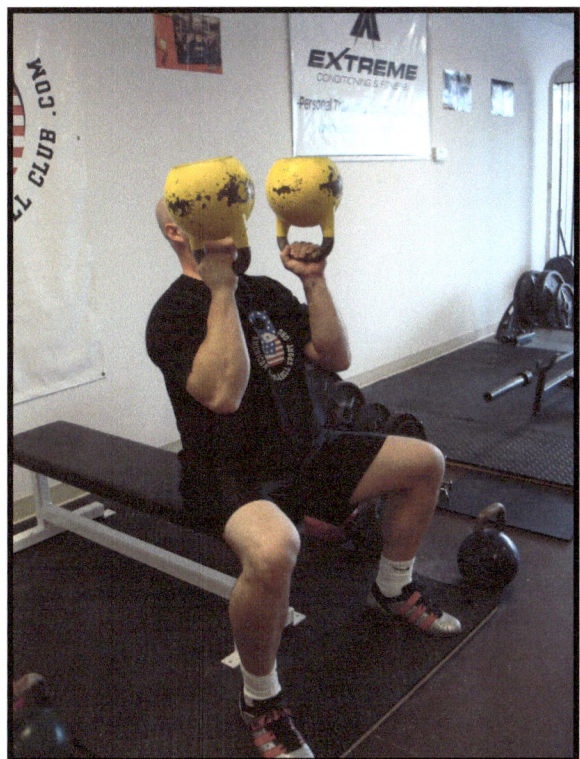
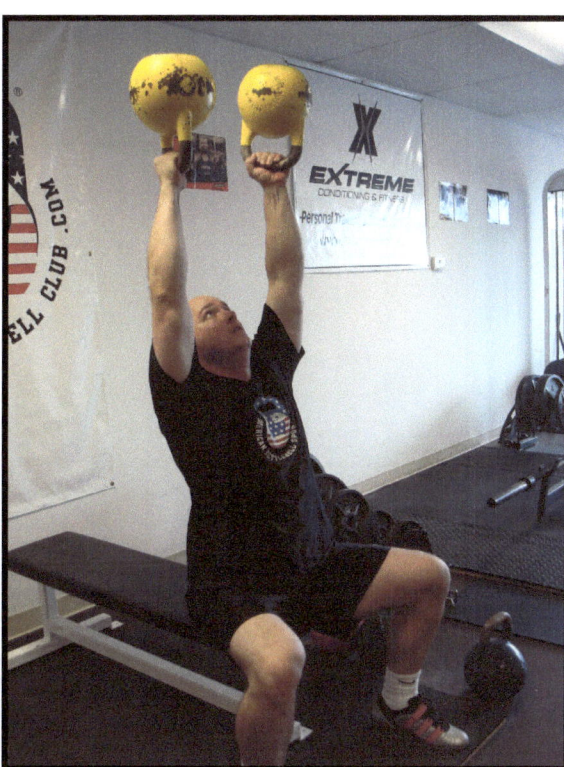

Bottom-Up Chair Press

Primary Muscles Worked

deltoids, triceps

Push Press

The push press is similar to the press with the main difference being an initial knee dip followed by a forceful straightening of the knees and hips to initiate the upward movement of the kettlebell. The initial knee dip throws the kettlebell into the air at which point you continue to press the bell with the arm to a proper lockout position. Drop the bell back to the rack position to complete the repetition.

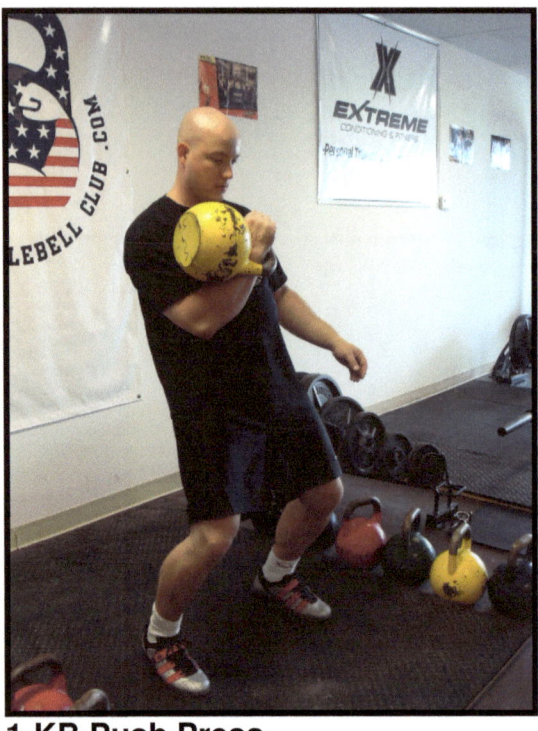
1-KB Push Press

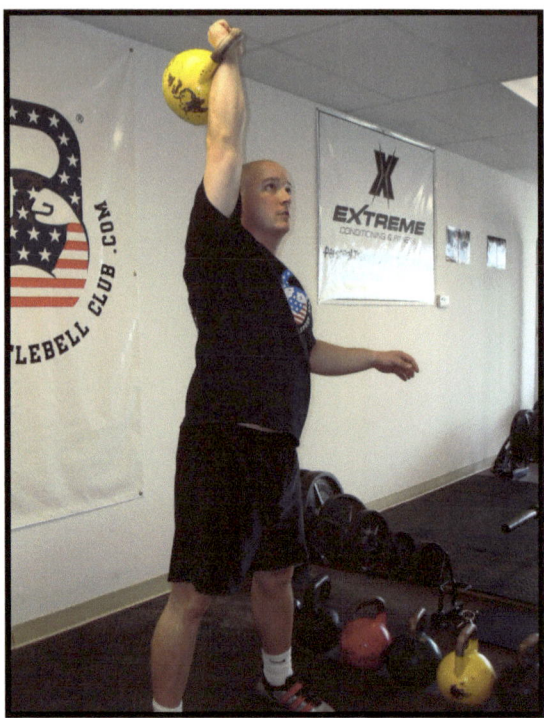

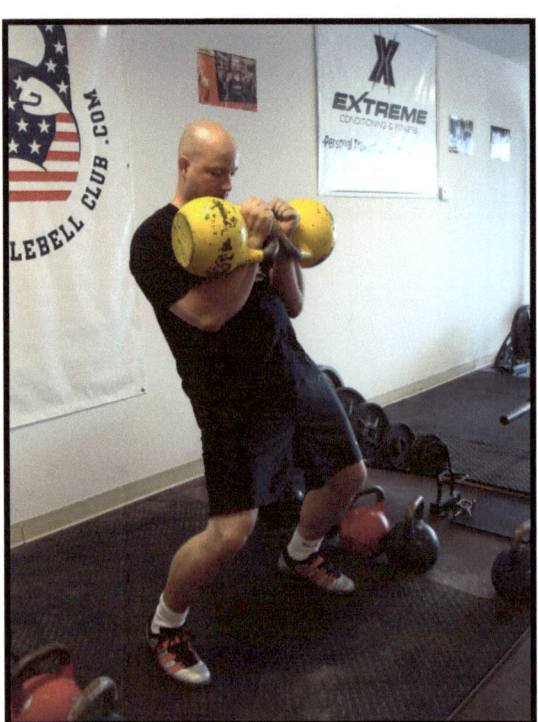
2-KB Push Press

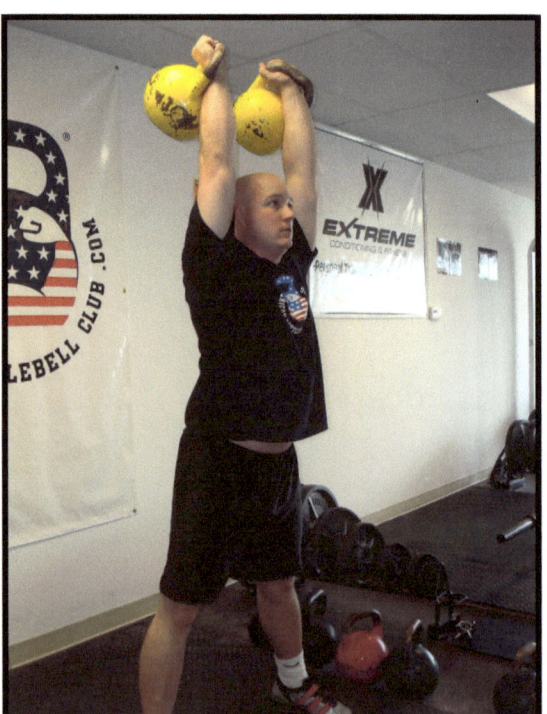

In the push press the RPMs will typically range from 4-16. Push presses may be performed with one or two kettlebells.

Variations

Bottom-Up Push Press

The bottom-up push press is performed by cleaning the kettlebell(s) into a bottom-up position then performing the push press. This will emphasize the grip in addition to the other muscle groups worked in the push press exercise.

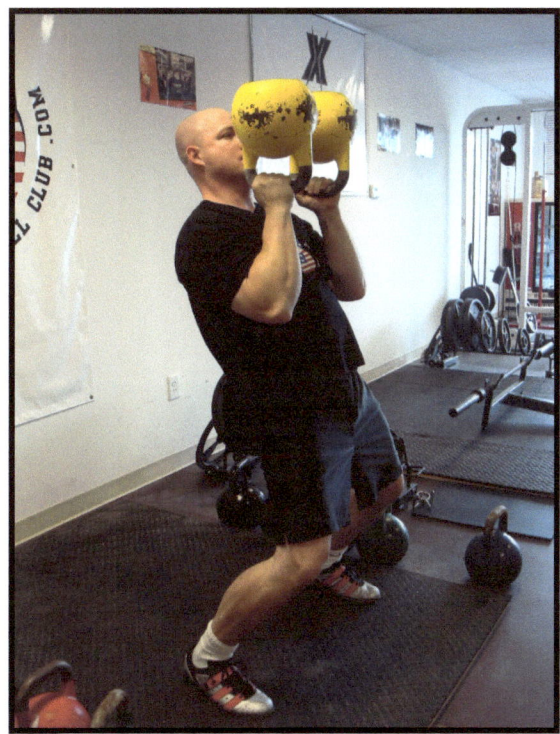
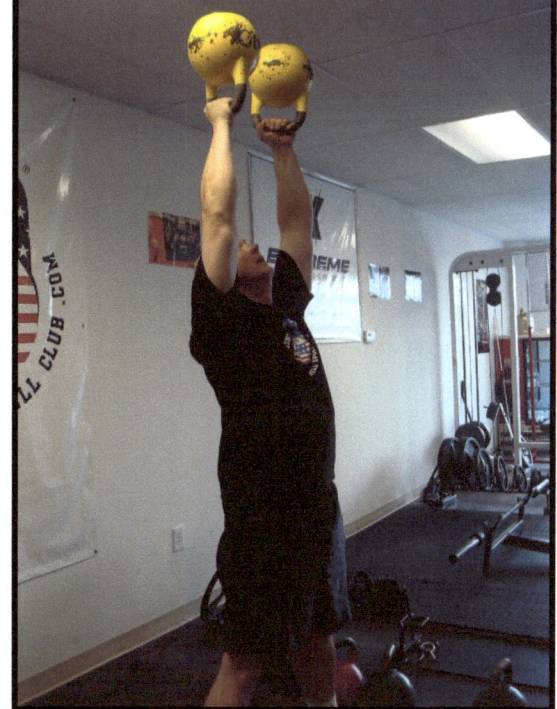

2-KB Bottom-Up Push Press

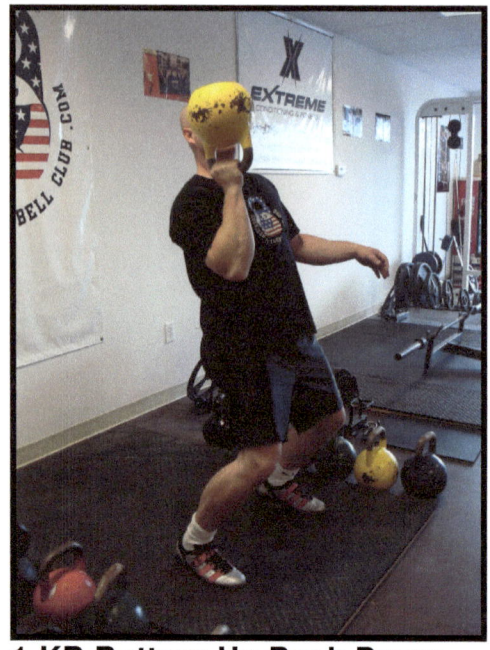 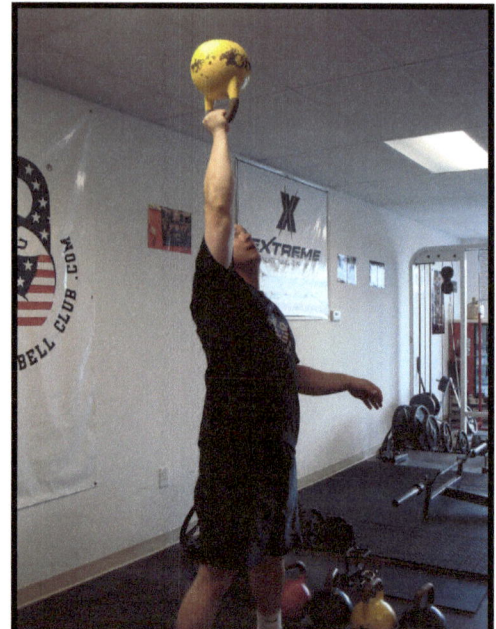

1-KB Bottom-Up Push Press

Primary Muscles Worked

quads, glutes, deltoids, triceps

Jerk

The jerk begins with the initial knee dip like the push press, however after the bell is sent into the air the lifter immediately drops into a second knee dip catching the bell with the arm fully extended and locked-out overhead.

At this point the lifter straightens the knees and hips to be fully extended into a true lockout position. The bell is dropped to the rack position to complete the repetition.

The two kettlebell jerk, sometimes called the short cycle jerk, is one of the lifts contested in the sport of kettlebell lifting and along with the snatch makes up what is known as the biathlon event.

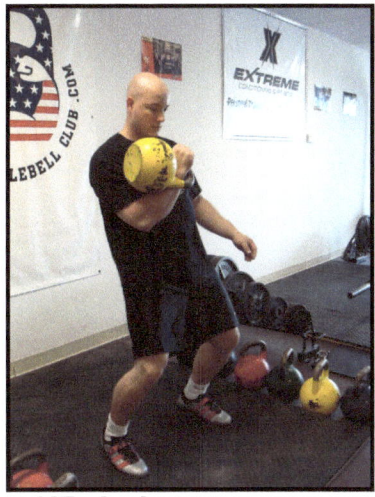 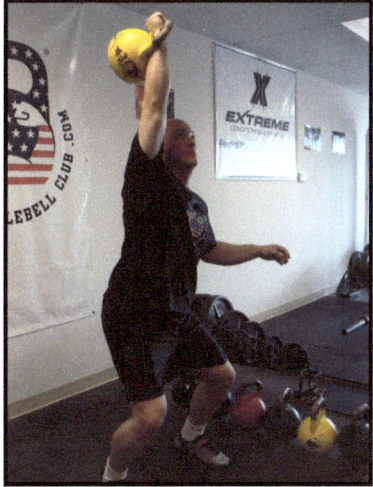 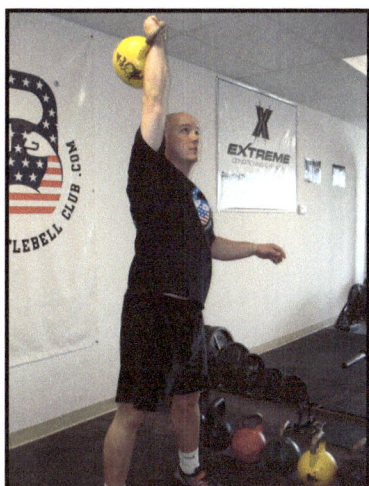

1-KB Jerk

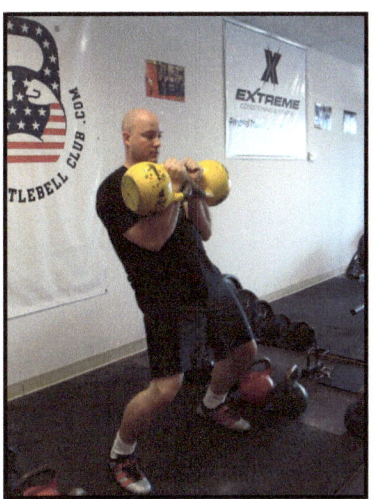 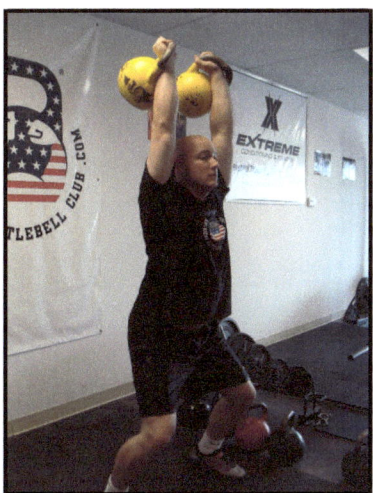 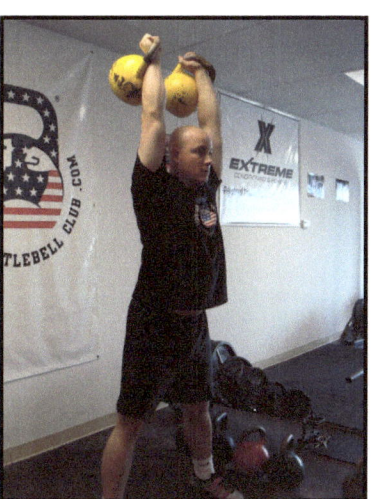

2-KB Jerk

In the jerk the RPMs will typically range from 4-16. Jerks may be performed with one or two kettlebells. The absolute world champion in the sport of kettlebell lifting, Ivan Denisov, has the world record in the jerk with 175 reps in 10:00 with a pair of 32kg kettlebells. That is 140 pounds with an average of 17-18 reps per minute or 24,500 pounds of work in one continuous set!

Primary Muscles Worked

quads, glutes, deltoids, triceps

Long Cycle

The long cycle exercise can be performed as a press, push press, or jerk. What makes this lift "long cycle" is that the clean is performed every repetition prior to the overhead phase of the exercise.

Due to this fact, the long cycle is probably the "biggest bang for your buck" in all of the traditional kettlebell lifts. If you only had 10-15 minutes to get a workout in, grab a kettlebell and perform the 1-arm long cycle without setting the bell down. I guarantee if you doubted my previous statement, you will agree with me whole-heartedly after this "abbreviated" workout!

The long cycle is performed by first doing a clean, then either pressing, push pressing or jerking the bell overhead. After the overhead phase is complete, re-clean the bell and perform the next overhead repetition.

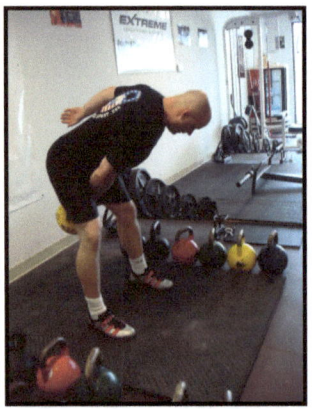 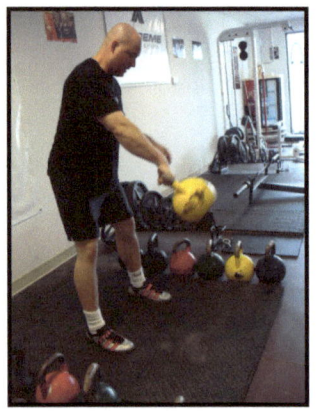 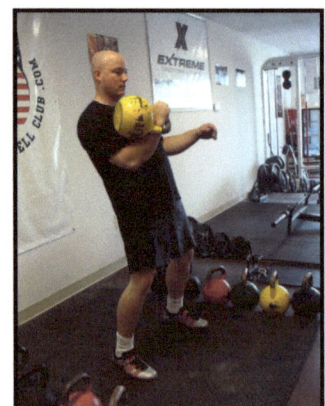

1-Arm Long Cycle Jerk

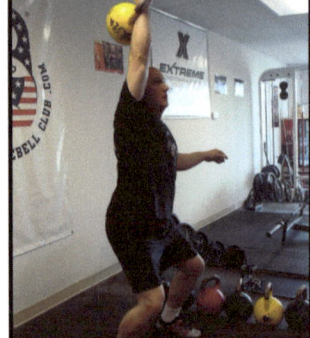 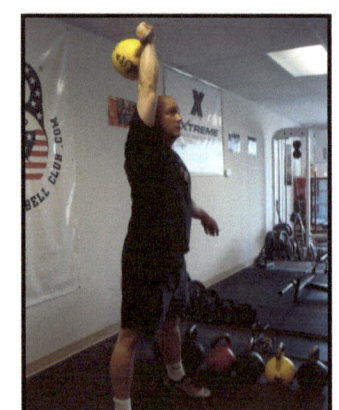

In the long cycle the RPMs will typically range from 4-10. Long cycle may be performed with one or two kettlebells. The two kettlebell variation is one of the contested lifts in the sport of kettlebell lifting and is its own event, separate from the biathlon. The great Ivan Denisov holds the world record in the long cycle event with 109 repetitions in 10:00 with a pair of 32kg bells.

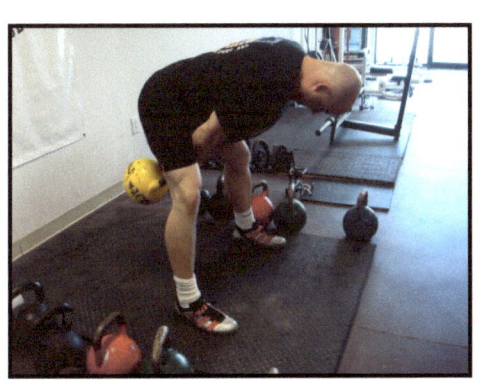 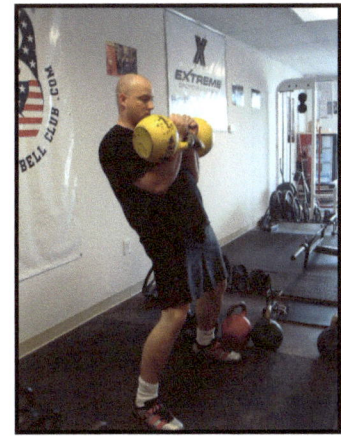 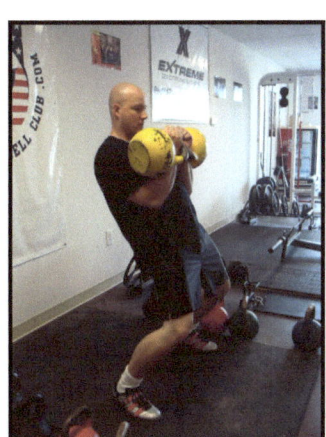

Long Cycle Clean and Jerk

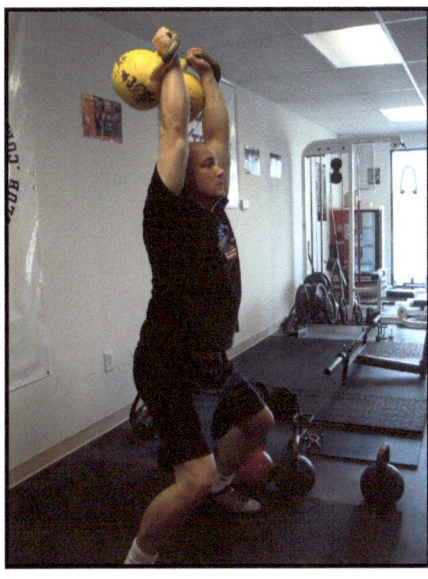 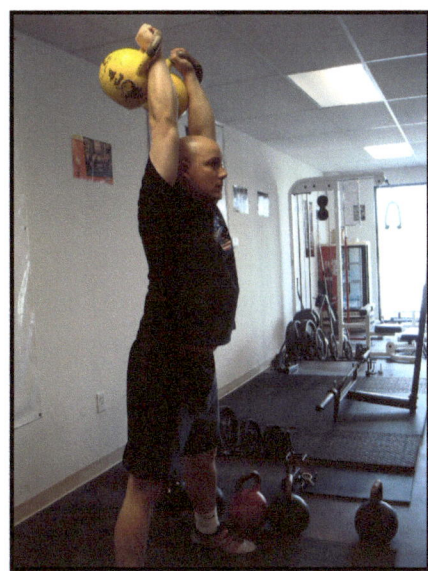

Variations

Bottom-Up Long Cycle

Bottom-up variations may be performed for the long cycle press and long cycle push press. I do not recommend performing any variation of the jerk bottom-up as it is too dynamic of a movement and the risks are too great while balancing a kettlebell upside down.

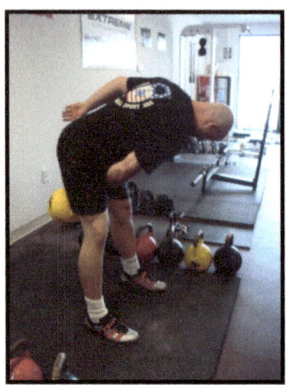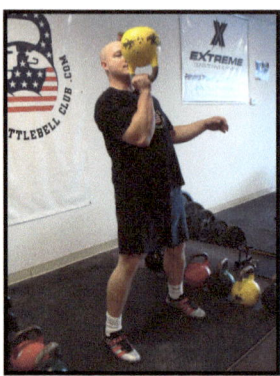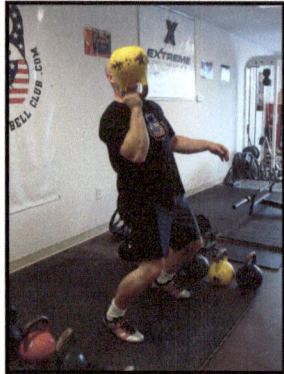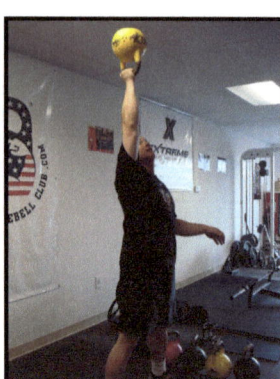

1-Arm Bottom-Up Long Cycle

Primary Muscles Worked

quads, hamstrings, glutes, lower back, upper back, deltoids, triceps, grip

Snatch

The snatch picks up where the swing leaves off. At the peak of the swing the snatch continues driving the bell overhead at which point the handle is "rotated around the bell" allowing the bell to come to rest in the overhead lockout position, identical to the overhead position of a press, push press, jerk, etc.

After the correct overhead fixation, roll the bell around the outside of the wrist and forearm by bending the elbow slightly and dropping the arm in front of the body. This is what is sometimes referred to as the "corkscrew" technique. Allow the bell to fall naturally and swing back between the legs. Once the bell totally decelerates reverse the movement and perform the next repetition.

It is very important to "follow the bell" with the eyes as in the swing. This will allow your back to stay in a neutral position. There is no need to arch the lower back as in the deadlift, barbell clean or barbell snatch, simply keep the lower back in a neutral position throughout the exercise.

Some flexion of the upper (thoracic) back may occur in the bottom part of the snatch during the swing back, this is fine. The snatch is one of the lifts contested in the sport of kettlebell lifting and along with the jerk makes up what is known as the biathlon.

The snatch is performed with one kettlebell, although in the 1984 Weightlifting Yearbook, it was reported that at one time the two kettlebell snatch was being considered for inclusion in the biathlon event.

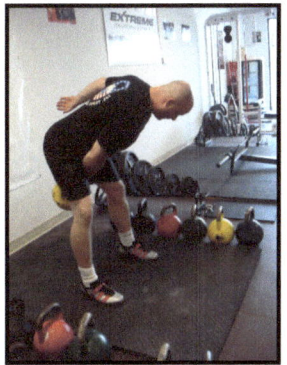 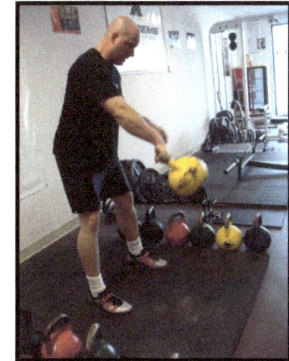 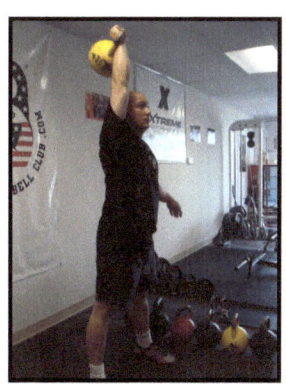

Snatch

The snatch is typically performed for 12-16 RPMs, although competitive lifters at the higher levels will approach 20-22 RPMs. Both Valery Fedorenko and current absolute world champion Ivan Denisov have performed 220 reps with the 32kb bell. That is 22 RPMs with a 70 pound kettlebell for 10:00 with only one hand switch. Try it and let me know how it goes!

Primary Muscles Worked

hamstrings, glutes, lower and upper back, deltoids, grip

Jumping Squats

Granted this is not exactly a kettlebell lift, but it is a lift that can help build your jerk numbers. Let me preface this exercise description with this warning, the jumping squat is an advanced exercise. If you are a kettlebell sport competitor looking for a tool to help raise your jerk or long cycle numbers, the jumping squat is an excellent choice. If you are training for fitness or are a beginner in the sport of kettlebell lifting, skip the jumping squat altogether.

The jumping squat is the equivalent of an explosive calf raise. The knees and hips go through a range of motion similar to that of the jerk. The exercise is a ¼ squat at most. Simply drop into a ¼ squat, explode up to the tips of the toes or to the point where the feet leave the ground altogether, and land back in the ¼ squat position.

Do not land with locked knees, simply drop into the next repetition and repeat until all repetitions are complete.

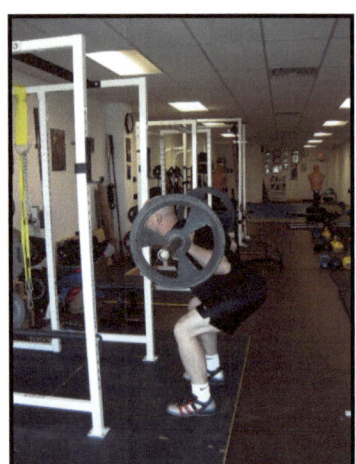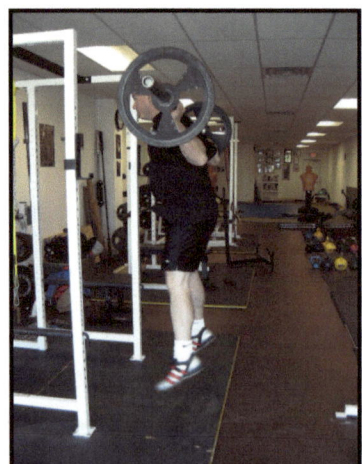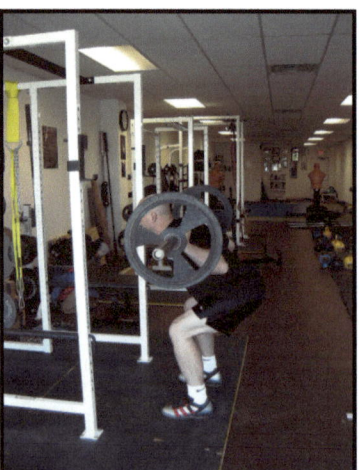

Jumping Squat, an advanced exercise to build the jerk

The jumping squat is typically performed for 2-3 sets of 30-50 repetitions. The weight will typically range from 185 lbs to 225 lbs for most athletes. However, I know some highly ranked lifters who have worked up to 315 lbs and more in this exercise!

Primary Muscles Worked

glutes, hamstrings, quadriceps, calves

Non-Traditional Exercises

There are a few exercises that are not considered "traditional exercises" in kettlebell lifting that I have found useful for my clients and athletes. For these exercises we typically perform a certain number of sets and repetitions as opposed to timed sets with designated RPMs.

These exercises are used primarily in lieu of a more traditional barbell or dumbbell exercise. The structure of the kettlebell adds a dimension that we do not get with the barbell or dumbbell variation.

Again, you may perform any exercise you choose with a kettlebell, the goal in writing this book was to introduce the traditional exercises, as well as certain non-traditional exercises and how we implement them at my training facility.

That being said, here are a few of the non-traditional exercises we feel have been beneficial to our training program.

Kettlebell Front Squat

Front squats are a fantastic variation of the squat. They allow the lifter to squat with a very upright torso, compared to a back squat, placing less stress on the lumbar spine. They provide excellent loading for the quadriceps as well.

The greatest challenge many of my lifters face is building the flexibility in the wrists to hold the barbell in the "clean" position at the chest. Considering we are not Olympic weightlifters, and the front squat is more of a variation than a staple in our training, we prefer alternatives that allow us to get the job done.

There are various harnesses and straps that may be attached to the bar to allow us to perform the exercise without reverting to the "folded arm" variation.

Another option we like is to perform a front squat after cleaning a pair of kettlebells to the chest. The only drawback to this exercise is that kettlebells do not offer incremental loading options.

Again, due to the fact that this is predominantly a supplementary exercise for my lifters, it is not that big of an issue. It is an easy to perform exercise that is particularly easy on those of us who posses wrists that are more "flexibility challenged" than others.

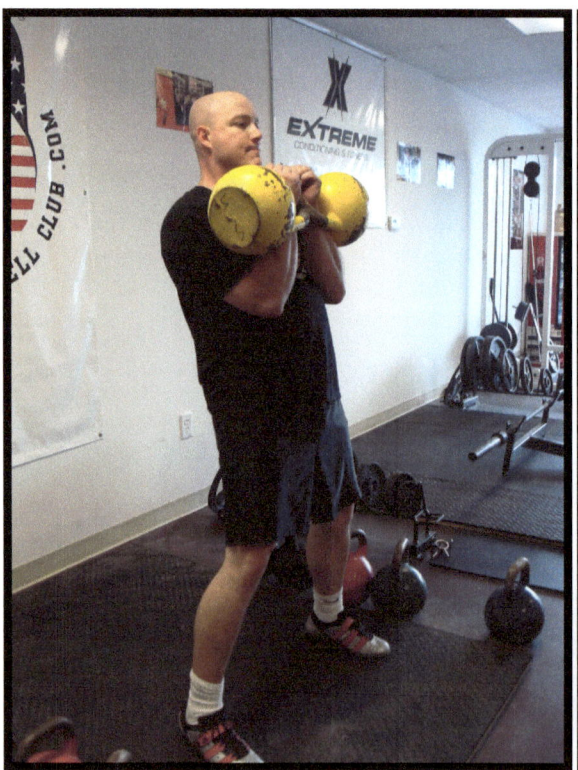 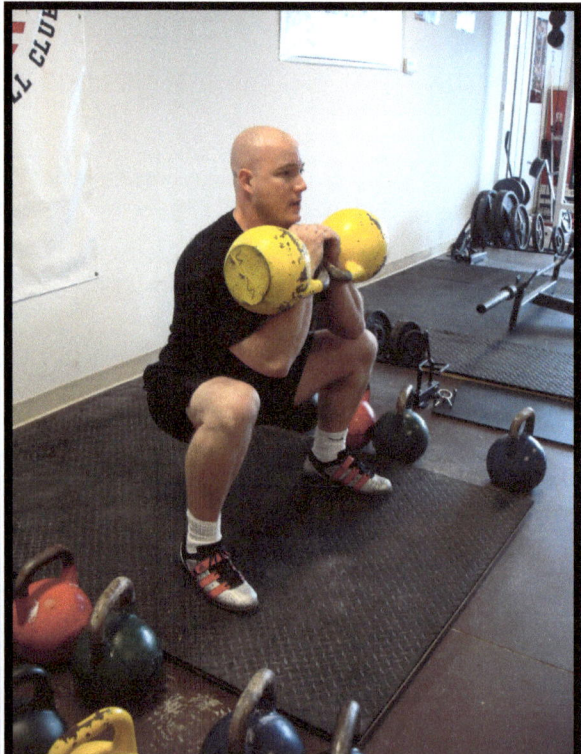

2-KB Front Squat

Primary Muscles Worked

quads, glutes, hamstrings, torso musculature, lower and upper back

Kettlebell Hammer Curl

I know, I know. Curls are for girls and bodybuilders. However, there is nothing wrong with having strong biceps when deadlifting or picking up heavy stones, plus I would rather have "muscular strong" arms over "skinny strong" arms any day of the week.

Hammer curls are an excellent choice as they work both the biceps and the forearms. By performing the hammer curl with a kettlebell, the wrist and grip are overloaded as well due to the nature of the suspended weight design of the bell.

To perform this exercise, hold a kettlebell with your palm facing the midline of the body and flex the elbow performing a typical biceps curl. Reverse the movement and repeat for the desired number of repetitions.

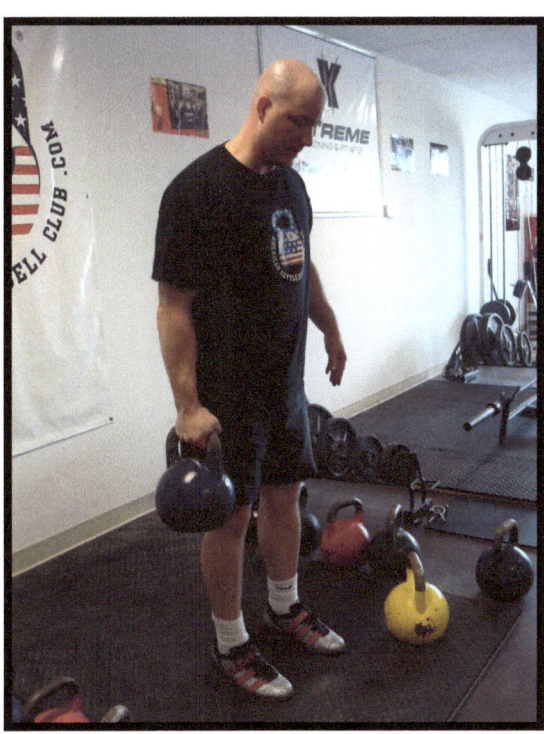 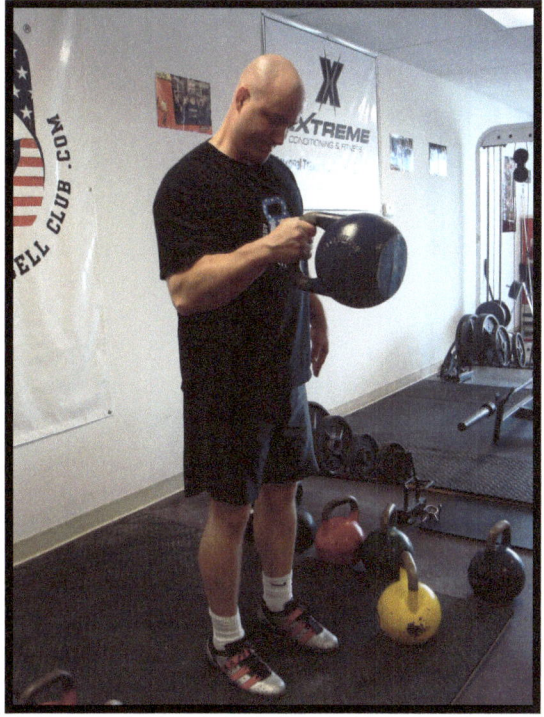

Kettlebell Hammer Curl

Primary Muscles Worked

biceps, brachialis, forearms, wrist, grip

Kettlebell Triceps Extension

Triceps are important for building bench press lockout strength. Most of the powerlifters that train with me perform many variations of the triceps extension exercise after benching and specific lockout work. Some of our lifters have experienced elbow pain due to all the extension work.

When we began adding the kettlebell extensions into our program they did not seem to stress the lifter's elbows as badly as the barbell and dumbbell variations. While we may not hold any all-time records in the bench press, we have a handful of lifters with some pretty solid numbers.

Malcom Gunter has an official bench press of 502 at a bodyweight of 198 lbs. That lift put him at #78 in Powerlifting USA magazine's Top 100 list in 2006.

David Cohn, an elite 114 class lifter who made #3 Powerlifting USA magazine's Top 100 list in 2007 with an 1100 total, has official bench press lifts of 275 at a bodyweight of 111 lbs and 305 at a bodyweight of 120 lbs at the time this book is being written. Both of these lifts were performed in a single-ply shirt. He's also made a solid 315 in training and has a bright lifting career ahead of him.

One of our novice lifters, Andre Cuadrado, made an easy 335 raw bench press at a bodyweight of 194 lbs. We are expecting big things from Andre as well as he is already closing in on a raw 400 bench in training.

All three of these guys perform a ton of kettlebell triceps extensions and credit them as one of the assistance exercises that really got their bench press moving.

To perform this lift lie down on the ground with a pair of kettlebells positioned on either side of your head. Grab the handles and explosively extend the elbows to fully lockout the arms. Lower the weights back to the starting position, allowing the bells to come to rest briefly on the ground and repeat for the desired number of repetitions.

The key is to allow the bells to rest on the ground, this makes the exercise a static overcome by dynamic movement. For more on the benefits of this type of training read almost any article authored by the great Louie Simmons of Westside Barbell. With a 502 bench press Malcom regularly works the 32kg bells for sets of 10 or so.

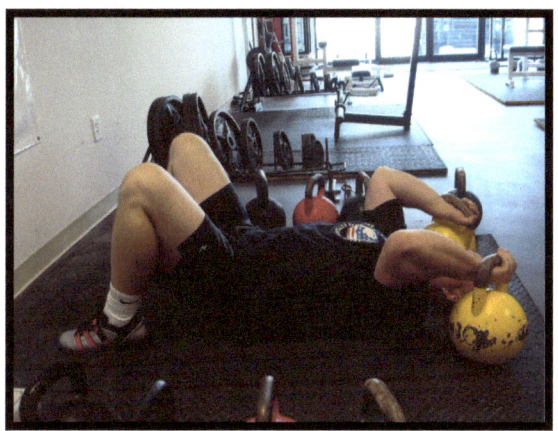 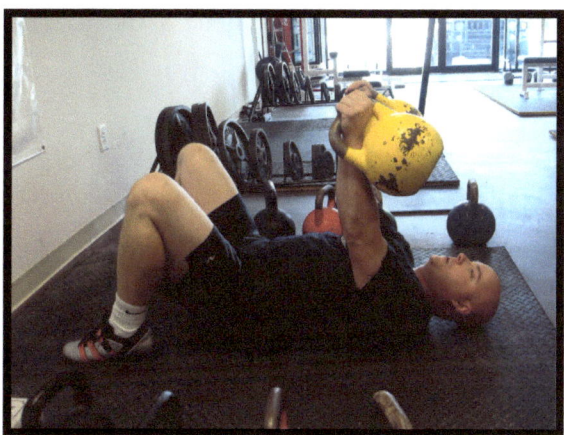

Kettlebell Triceps Extension

Primary Muscles Worked

triceps

There you have it, eleven exercises and variations that make up the bulk of the kettlebell training performed by my athletes, clients, and me at my training facility.

In the next chapter I will present numerous sample templates to demonstrate how we put these exercises together in our training program and hopefully give you some ideas on how you may build your own training plan or add to the one you currently follow.

Chapter 4
Training Templates

The bulk of the athletes I train come to me with the goal of improving strength and power. This group is made up of football players, powerlifters, and people who just want to be strong and in great shape.

I work with athletes from other sports (such as wrestling, tennis, golf, adventure racing, water-skiing, bodybuilding, figure/fitness, mountain climbing, martial arts, baseball, and basketball), law enforcement agents, fire fighters, business owners and professionals, as well as many general fitness enthusiasts who are looking for a challenging way to enhance their personal fitness program.

In this chapter I will present some of the general training templates that we have implemented with some of my athletes and clients as well as some of the templates I have learned about through my experiences as an AKC coach regarding the training of the kettlebell sport competitor.

Keep in mind these are general templates and the goal is to give you ideas of how you may build your own training program specific to your needs. These templates are not the be-all end-all of kettlebell lifting but rather a guide to introduce you to some of the methods I have learned in my experience with kettlebells and kettlebell training.

If you want to talk more in-depth about training plans please feel free to contact me through my website at: **www.extreme-fitness.org** or through email at: **scott@extreme-fitness.org**.

Training Templates for Strength and Sport

As I mentioned previously, the bulk of the work I do is strength training for athletes and clients in strength and power related sports or disciplines, therefore this section will contain most of the information I've put together regarding training templates and program development.

Kettlebells can be a very effective tool in the tool box of the strength and conditioning professional and athlete. While I do not believe they are of much benefit regarding maximal strength or explosive strength, I feel they are extremely valuable for general physical preparation (GPP) as well as weak point training.

In speaking with Valery Fedorenko at the 2008 American Kettlebell Club Classic in Las Vegas, he expressed to me that a powerlifter or strength athlete can best use kettlebells to improve recovery and GPP. Essentially, they get you in shape to lift.

In powerlifting it is important to be as strong as possible all over. However, at least in the lifters I train and train with at my gym, the shoulders, triceps, lower back, abs and hamstrings tend to be problem areas. Various kettlebell lifts can be quite useful when performing extra work and GPP for these muscle groups. Louie Simmons has written extensively on the importance of GPP for powerlifters, so I will not go into it here.

As mentioned in the previous chapter, the lifts we focus on are mostly the traditional lifts done for timed sets performed at the end of the training session. In addition to his articles on GPP, Louie Simmons has also written about the value of timed sets of exercises when performing lifts using the repeated effort method in his training and that of his lifters.

One comment that stuck out to me is that it is important to hold the weight the entire set as this keeps constant tension on the muscles being worked. This is very similar to the importance of not setting the kettlebell down during the performance of the kettlebell exercises we recommend. If you take the liberty of setting the bell down at will, you will lose out on a valuable aspect of this training. Usually only one set of one or two kettlebell exercises are performed.

We typically work in the range of a 2-3 minute set, but will sometimes push it up to 5 minutes when conditioning is a priority. We typically begin at a slower repetition per minute pace with the kettlebell lifts and then begin increasing the RPMs as the workouts become easier.

The following is a list of kettlebell exercises we tend to focus on.

Swing
Clean
Snatch
Press
Chair press
Push Press
Jerk
Long Cycle (Clean & Press, Clean & Push-Press or Clean & Jerk)

Swings are performed in a continuous pace so there is not a specific RPM designated for this exercise. For snatches we typically work in the range of 12-16 RPMs. For presses and jerks begin around 4-5 RPMs and build up to 16 RPMs. For long cycle begin around 4-5 RPMs and build up to 10 RPMs.

Newer lifters will start with 16kg bells then build up to 24kg and eventually 32kg. It is wise to progress to a higher RPM for longer sets before moving up in weight. My training partner Derrick, a 242 class lifter, found out the hard way.

When he began adding timed sets of long cycle into his training program his very first workout he tried to go 3 minutes with a pair of 24kg kettlebells. He figured that since he has bench pressed in the mid-high 400's how hard could 3 minutes with 106 pounds really be?

Well he just about made the 3 minute set and very soon after he deposited the pulled pork sandwich he had about 6 hours earlier at lunch in the bathroom of my gym. He moved down to the 16kg bells for his next training session!

Let's take a look at the lifters I mentioned in the previous chapter that I train and train with and how we work kettlebells into the training plan.

Malcom Gunter is a bench-only lifter who has made a 502 pound bench in the 198 pound weight class. This lift put him at #78 in Powerlifting USA's Top 100 lifters for the 198 weight class in 2006. Malcom is currently making the transition to a full meet lifter and is using kettlebells to help bring up his lower back and hamstring strength for the squat and deadlift as well as the benefit he's experienced with his bench press through long cycle, presses and extensions.

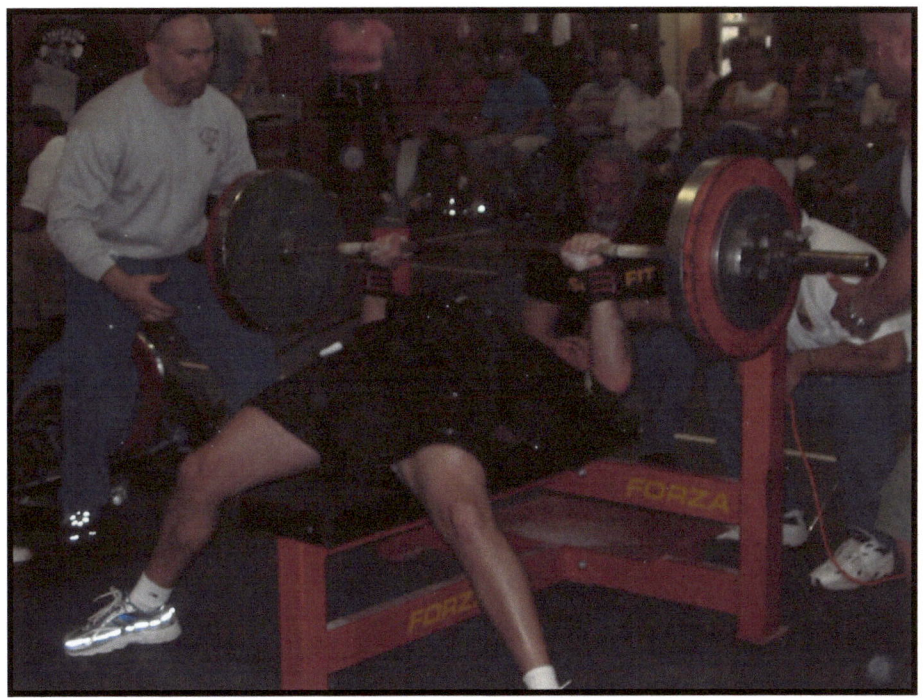
Malcom Gunter

David Cohn is a full meet lifter in the 114 and 123 pound weight classes. In the 114 pound class David has the following best lifts; squat 400, bench press 275, deadlift 430 and an elite total of 1100 all at 111 pounds bodyweight.

David's 1100 pound total put him at #2 out of all men in 2007 Powerlifting USA's Top 100 lifters for the 114 weight class. In the 123 pound weight class David has the following best lifts; squat 405, bench press 305, deadlift 405 and a Master Class total of 1115.

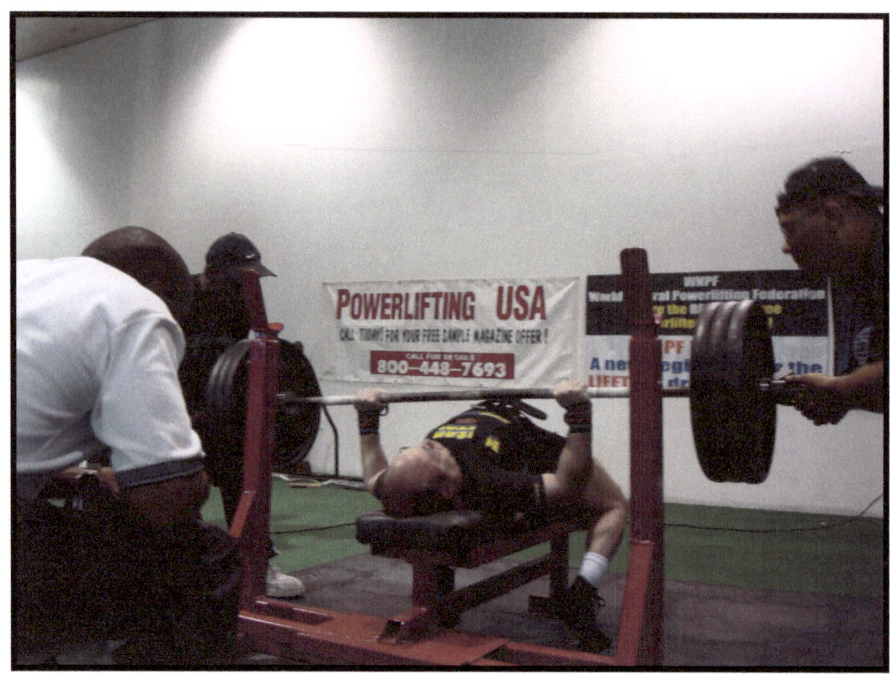
David Cohn

Andre Cuadrado is a novice full meet lifter in the 198 pound weight class. Andre lifts in the raw division and after only 2 meets has posted best lifts of a 500 pound squat, a bench press of 335 pounds, a deadlift of 545 pounds, and a Class 1 raw total of 1360 at a bodyweight of 194 lbs.

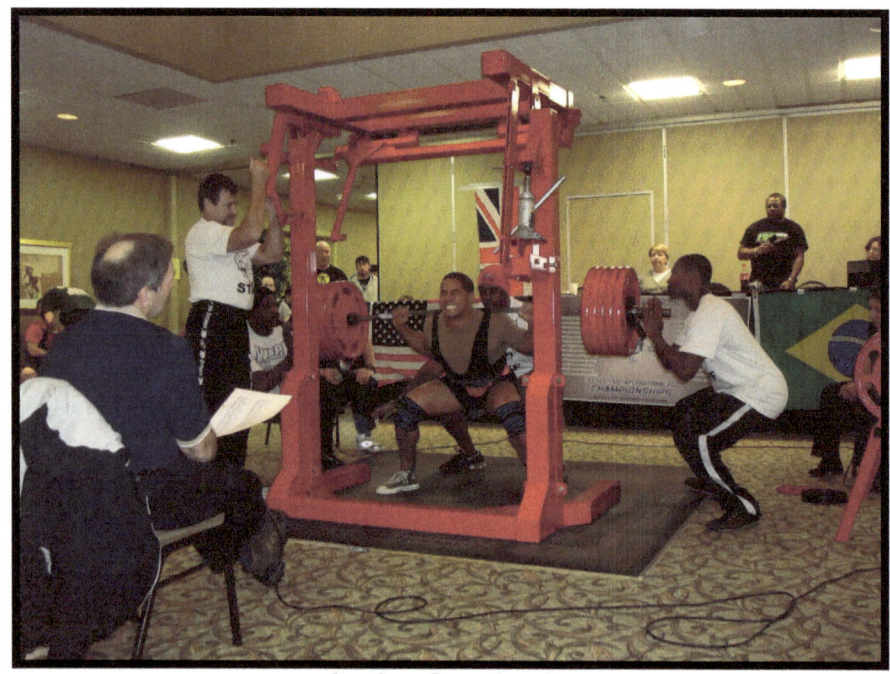
Andre Cuadrado

In addition to the powerlifters I train with and coach, I work with conventional sport athletes as well.

Cory Clemons graduated from Georgia Southern University in 2007 where he played outside linebacker. Cory came to me in January 2008 to begin training for his school's pro-day and Scout Camp regional combine and is currently getting ready for some Arena Football League tryouts.

Some of Cory's preliminary test numbers were as follows:

Height - 6'0"
Weight - 237 pounds
40 yard dash - 4.85 seconds
Vertical jump - 29"
Bench press 225 pounds - 16 repetitions
Squat one rep max - 535 pounds
Bench press one rep max - 335 pounds

We determined that Cory's lower back was extremely weak and a limiting factor in his speed, strength and power. We performed many of the same lifts in Cory's training program that he performed while training throughout his college career. The only new exercises I introduced were kettlebell swings and snatches with the goal of strengthening Cory's weak lower back.

Four months later Cory made the following improvements in his tests:

Weight - 247 pounds (10 pound increase)
40 yard dash - 4.71 seconds (0.14 second improvement)
Vertical jump - 39.5" (10.5" improvement)
Bench press 225 pounds - 23 reps (a 7 rep improvement)
Squat one rep max - 600 pounds (65 pound increase)
Bench press one rep max - 405 (70 pound increase)

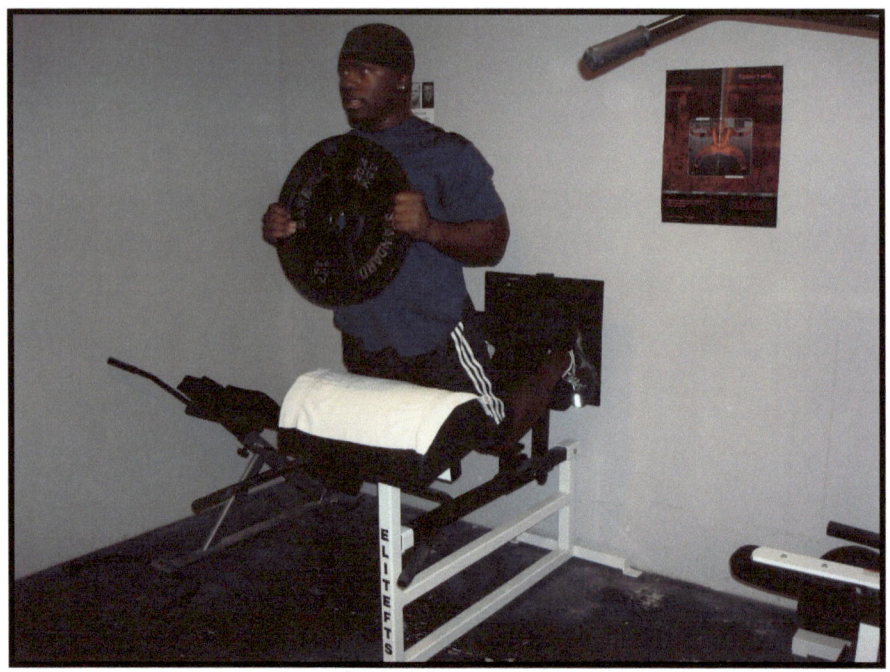
Cory Clemons

The following are some of the training templates my lifters and I utilize at various times throughout the year.

Westside Barbell Inspired Training Template – this is the most commonly used training plan at my gym. There is some variance for each individual lifter at different times of the year, especially when training for a meet or specific goal.

Monday – Max Effort Squat/Deadlift
1. Max Effort exercise, we rotate between a squat, good morning and deadlift variation for a 1RM
2. Supplementary lift, usually a posterior chain exercise
3. Abdominal exercise
4. Kettlebell swings, jerks or long cycle – 2-5 minutes
5. Sled or prowler work

Wednesday – Max Effort Bench Press
1. Max Effort exercise, we rotate between different bench press variations for a 1RM
2. Triceps lifts, usually one or two exercises

3. Lats/upper back, usually one or two exercises
   4. Kettlebell snatches or presses– 2-5 minutes
   5. Sled or prowler work

Friday – Dynamic Effort Squat/Deadlift
   1. Box Squats, waving between 50%-60% of a 1RM over 3 weeks for 8-12 sets of 2 reps
   2. Speed Deadlifts, waving between 50%-60% of a 1RM over 3 weeks for 5-8 sets of 1 rep
   3. Supplementary lift, usually a posterior chain exercise
   4. Abdominal exercise
   5. Kettlebell swings, jerks or long cycle – 2-5 minutes
   6. Sled or prowler work

Sunday – Dynamic Effort Bench Press
   1. Speed bench, usually 55% of a 1RM for 8-9 sets of 3 reps
   2. Triceps lifts, usually one or two exercises
   3. Lats/upper back, usually one or two exercises
   4. Kettlebell snatches or presses – 2-5 minutes
   5. Sled or prowler work

Basic "Power-building" Template – we call this the 4x4, four lifts over four days and draws its inspiration from Jim Wendler of Elite Fitness Systems and his incredibly simplistic, yet incredibly effective approach to strength training. You may also rotate this over three days per week if you need more recovery time. Want to get strong and get in shape? Stick with the basics and work them hard!

Monday – Squat
   1. Squat (heavy)
   2. Squat assistance lift
   3. Abdominal exercise
   4. Jerks or long cycle – 2-5 minutes

Wednesday – Bench Press
   1. Bench press (heavy)
   2. Bench assistance lift
   3. Upper back

    4. Swings or snatch – 2-5 minutes

Friday – Deadlift
1. Deadlift (heavy)
2. Deadlift assistance lift
3. Abdominal exercise
4. Jerks or long cycle – 2-5 minutes

Sunday – Military Press
1. Military press (heavy)
2. Close grip bench (light)
3. Lats
4. Swings or snatch – 2-5 minutes

The Bodybuilder – This is a variation of the power-building template for someone looking for more specific muscle size performed over four training days.

Monday
1. Squat (moderate intensity, high volume)
2. 1-leg squat or lunge
3. Calves
4. Abs
5. Jerk or long cycle – 2-5 minutes

Wednesday
1. Bench press (moderate intensity, high volume)
2. Horizontal pull (row variation)
3. Biceps
4. Swings or snatch – 2-5 minutes

Friday
1. Deadlift (moderate intensity, high volume)
2. Lower back
3. Traps
4. Abs
5. Jerk or long cycle – 2-5 minutes

Sunday

1. Military press (moderate intensity, high volume)
2. Vertical pull (pullups or pulldowns)
3. Triceps
4. Swings or snatch – 2-5 minutes

Powerlifting and Kettlebell Purist Template – no fluff, just the basic lifts for the powerlifting and kettlebell sport enthusiast. Perform the jerk and snatch as you would in competition, the jerk is performed with two kettlebells and only one hand switch in the snatch.

You may substitute the long cycle with two kettlebells for the jerk and snatch if you prefer the long cycle over the biathlon event in kettlebell sport. If you are prioritizing the kettlebell lifts perform them before the barbell lifts.

Monday
1. Squat (heavy)
2. Bench press (light)
3. Jerk – 5-7 minutes
4. Snatch – 6-8 minutes
5. Abdominal exercise

Wednesday
1. Bench press (heavy)
2. Deadlift (moderate-moderately heavy)
3. Jerk – 5-7 minutes
4. Snatch – 6-8 minutes
5. Abdominal exercise

Friday
1. Squat (light)
2. Bench press (moderate)
3. Jerk – 5-7 minutes
4. Snatch – 6-8 minutes
5. Abdominal exercise

I love my kettlebells but I don't want to ditch my barbells… just yet. This four day training plan is similar to the power-building template only with more emphasis on kettlebell lifts. You determine the length of sets, RPMs, and weight based on your experience level.

Monday
1. Kettlebell press
2. Double kettlebell clean
3. Double kettlebell chair press
4. Kettlebell swing
5. Abdominal exercise

Wednesday
1. Kettlebell press
2. Double kettlebell jerk
3. Barbell back squat
4. Pull ups
5. Kettlebell snatch

Friday
1. 1-arm long cycle
2. 1-arm kettlebell chair press
3. Dips
4. Kettlebell swing
5. Abdominal exercise

Sunday
1. Double kettlebell jerk
2. Pullups
3. Barbell bench press
4. Barbell deadlift
5. Kettlebell snatch

Templates for the Kettlebell Purist and Sport Lifter

Kettlebell Sport Beginner – this template requires one training session per day and five to six training days per week and is good for the beginner. Take one or two days off.

Day one of the template should be a test day in which you try to go a full 10:00 in the competition lifts. Start with light bells and move up to your competition weight when you can max out the time with a fairly high RPM with the lighter bells.

The remaining days will require you to perform one set of 5:00-7:00 minutes with your target RPM. Once you can hit 7:00 fairly consistently at the target RPM, add 1 RPM and start over always using day one as a test day.

Monday (Test Day)
1. Jerk: goal is 10:00 with your target RPM (for beginners start around 4-5 RPM, move up to the next weight when you can get 8-10 RPM for the full 10:00)
2. Snatch: goal is 10:00 (5:00 per hand with one hand switch) with your target RPM (for beginners start around 12-14 RPM, move up to the next weight when you can get 16-20 RPM for the full 10:00)
3. Running: easy jog/run for 20:00-30:00

Tuesday – Saturday (Training Days)
1. Jerk: goal is 5:00-7:00 with your target RPM, be sure to add 1 RPM when you hit 7:00 consistently.
2. Snatch: goal is 6:00-8:00 (3:00-4:00 per hand with one hand switch) with your target RPM, be sure to add 1 RPM when you hit 8:00 consistently.
3. Running: easy jog/run for 20:00-30:00

If your goal is to compete in the long cycle simply substitute the long cycle clean and jerk for the jerk and drop the snatches. Keep the running for general conditioning.

Kettlebell Sport Amateur – This template is for the amateur competitive lifter. It requires one training session per day and six training days per week. At this level the lifter should be training with 24kg kettlebells. As in the beginner template day one is a "test day".

Monday (Test Day)
1. Jerk: goal 10:00
2. Snatch: goal 10:00 (5:00 per hand with one hand switch)

Supplementary Exercises
1. 1-arm jerk w/32kg bell: build up to 1 set of 10-20 reps per arm
2. Swing w/32kg bell: build up to 1 set of 30-50 reps per arm
3. Jumping squats w/185-225 lbs: 2-3 sets of 30-50 reps*
4. Running: easy jog/run for 20:00-30:00

Jumping squats are an advanced exercise and only need to be implemented as a means of raising the numbers in the jerk for the higher level amateur lifter.

Tuesday – Saturday (Training Days)
1. Jerk: goal is 5:00-7:00
2. Snatch: goal is 6:00-8:00 (3:00-4:00 per hand with one hand switch)

Supplementary Exercises
1. 1-arm jerk w/32kg bell: build up to 1 set of 10-20 reps per arm
2. Swing w/32kg bell: build up to 1 set of 30-50 reps per arm
3. Jumping squats w/185-225 lbs: 2-3 sets of 30-50 reps
4. Running: easy jog/run for 20:00-30:00

If your goal is to compete in the long cycle simply substitute the long cycle clean and jerk for the jerk and drop the snatches. For supplementary work replace the 1-arm jerk and swing with the 1-arm long cycle and keep the jumping squats and the running.

Kettlebell Sport Professional – this template is for the fulltime professional lifter who is looking to move from a Master of Sport (MS) lifter classification to a Master of Sport International (MSIC) lifter classification.

This training plan requires two training sessions per day (one morning and one afternoon) and six training days per week. This is not an exact template a professional lifter would use, but rather some ideas that I picked up from Coach Fedorenko's presentation at my coaching certification I attended.

This template is for informational purposes only, since there are not very many lifters, if any at all, in this country ready for such a training plan at this time. Day one of the training week is still used as a "test day".

Sample Professional Training Schedule

a.m. Training Session
1. Snatch w/32kg: 1 set of 6:00-8:00 (go for a 10:00 set on the test day)
2. 1-arm jerk w/40kg: 1 set per arm
3. Swing w/40kg: 2 sets of 50 reps per arm
4. Running: easy run for 20:00-30:00

p.m. Training Session
1. snatch w/32kg: 1 set of 6:00-8:00
2. double jerk w/32kg: 5 sets of 5:00 at target RPM (go for a 10:00 set on the test day)
3. 1-arm jerk w/40kg: 1 set per arm
4. Swing w/40kg: 2 sets of 50 reps per arm
5. Jumping squats: 3 sets of 50 reps

I'm training for fitness not sport! – this template is perfect for someone who wants superior fitness training with kettlebells but isn't looking to compete or even train like a kettlebell sport athlete.

Begin with a light weight bell and the lowest RPMs for each lift. Build the RPMs and duration of each exercise before progressing to a heavier bell. Perform this workout three to four days per week. This is inspired by the WKC Kettlebell Fitness Program.

Warm up: joint mobility and light kettlebell swings

1. Kettlebell front squat: 10-30 reps; rest 0:30-2:00
2. Pick one (1-arm press, 1-arm push press, or 1-arm jerk): 1:00-3:00 per arm; rest 0:30-2:00
3. Pick one (1-arm clean, 1-arm snatch): 1:00-3:00 per arm; rest 0:30-2:00
4. Pick one (1-arm long cycle clean and press, 1-arm long cycle clean and push press, 1-arm long cycle clean and jerk): 1:00-3:00 per arm, rest 0:30-2:00
5. Repeat the above cycle 1-2 more times depending on your fitness level

Finisher: finish with 1-arm swings and abs – you choose the sets and reps.

Cool down: relaxation exercises and stretching.

If you want additional work there is nothing wrong with supplementing some cardiovascular work such as running, biking or rowing into this program.

There you have it. Nine sample templates that will hopefully get the gears turning in your head so that you may come up with some effective training plans of your own.

Remember, master the basic technique and lifts, it will pay huge dividends when moving on to more advanced training plans.

Conclusion

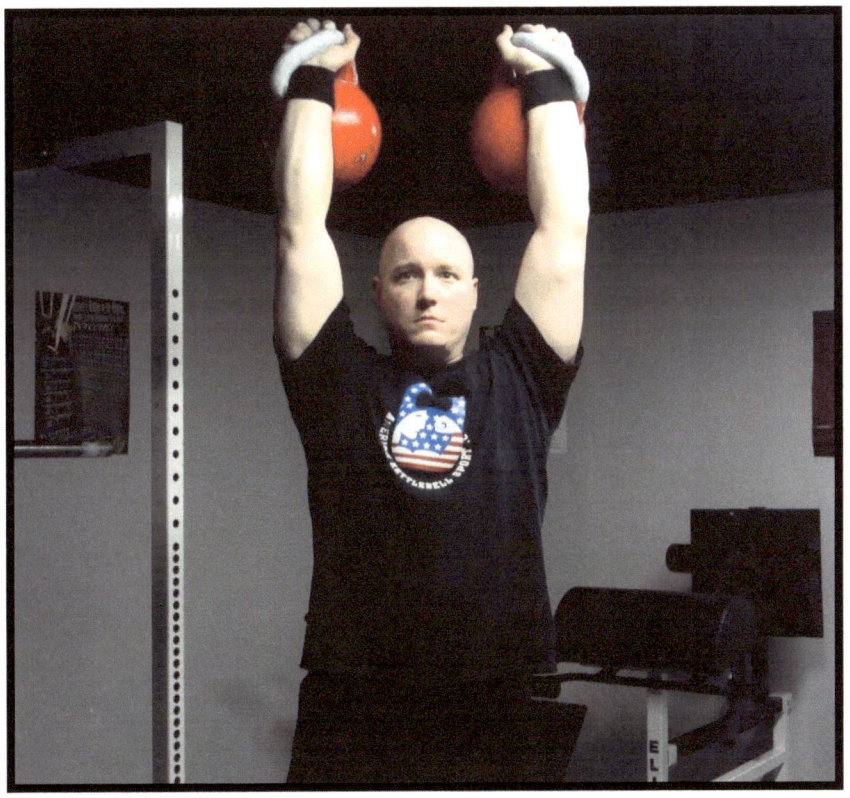

This book was written in order to present traditional kettlebell lifting methods and techniques and how to incorporate them into a training plan for sport, strength and fitness. In addition, I wanted to provide information pertaining to the history of kettlebells as well as sample training templates and ideas on how to incorporate kettlebells into your personal training program.

Kettlebells can be a valuable tool for sport, strength and fitness training. While they are not required to improve strength, speed, athleticism and fitness, my experience has shown me that they can contribute very well to those areas. Remember to build your training around the basics, but as you advance do not be afraid to experiment with new ideas and methods.

It is my sincerest hope that you found value in this book and that it has opened your mind to some new ideas and methods of training. I wish you the best of luck in your training program and hope you experience incredible gains and excellent health as a result.

Now, let's get in the gym and get to work!

In Strength, Health and Fitness,

Scott Shetler

About the Author

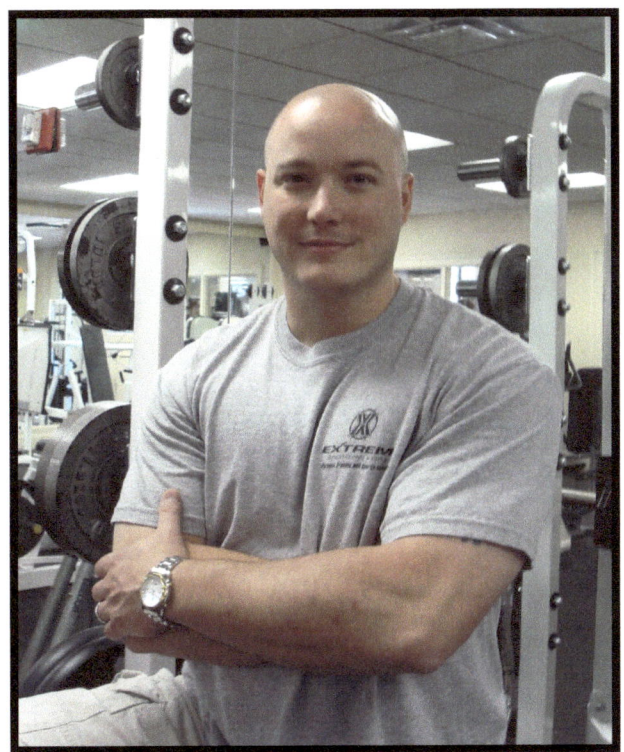

Scott Shetler

Scott is the owner of the Atlanta Barbell & Kettlebell Club and Extreme Conditioning and Fitness sport and fitness training. Scott trains athletes and general fitness enthusiasts alike, and has competed in both powerlifting and kettlebell sport. He is certified through the NSCA and is a Master Kettlebell Trainer through the American Kettlebell Club (AKC) and World Kettlebell Club (WKC) able to certify and license kettlebell instructors.

For more information please visit Scott on the web at **www.extreme-fitness.org** or contact him via email at **scott@extreme-fitness.org.**

References

1984 Weightlifting Yearbook. Translated by Andrew Charniga. Sportivny Press.

Caestus: The Extreme Girevoy Sport Records Blog. "Russian Girevoy Sport History." "Girevoy Sport Competition History 2." **caestuspalestra.wordpress.com**, 2008.

Fedorenko, Valery. Kettlebell Fitness Manual of World Kettlebell Club. World Kettlebell Club, 2008.

World Kettlebell Club. Lifter Ranking Tables. **www.worldkettlebellclub.com**.

Other Titles by the Author

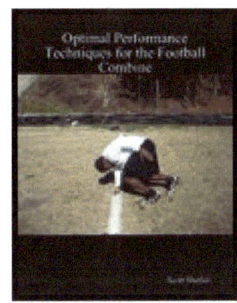

Optimal Performance Techniques for the Football Combine

This book teaches the optimal techniques for football combine performance enhancement. In addition the book discusses some effective strength training exercises as well as sample training templates. Do you want to drop 0.2 seconds off your 40 yd dash and add 2" to your vertical immediately? If so you need this book!

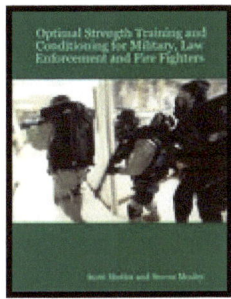

Optimal Strength Training and Conditioning for Military, Law Enforcement and Fire Fighters

This book presents the optimal methods of strength training and conditioning for those in the military, law enforcement, and fire fighting professions. If your job requires superior fitness get this book!

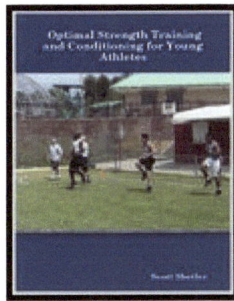

Optimal Strength Training and Conditioning for Young Athletes

A simple approach to the implementation of optimal strength training and conditioning methods for young athletes. You need to learn to crawl before you can walk. Don't overlook the basics, get this book and get started correctly!

For more information about our other products including training and consulting services, DVD's, books, t-shirts, customized supplement and meal plans, please visit us on the web at: **www.extreme-fitness.org**

For more information on becoming a Certified/Licensed Kettlebell Instructor contact Scott at: **scott@extreme-fitness.org**.

To register for our newsletter and receive free sport and fitness training tips and information, please email us at: **scott@extreme-fitness.org** and type "newsletter" in the subject line of the email.

www.ingramcontent.com/pod-product-compliance
Lightning Source LLC
Chambersburg PA
CBHW041552220426
43666CB00002B/43